Sugar Busters!®
for Kids

Sugar Busters!®
for Kids

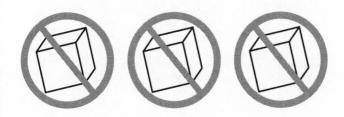

Samuel S. Andrews, M.D.

Morrison C. Bethea, M.D.

Luis A. Balart, M.D.

H. Leighton Steward

Ballantine Books • New York

A Ballantine Book
Published by The Ballantine Publishing Group

www.ballantinebooks.com
www.sugarbusters.com

Library of Congress Cataloging-in-Publication Data
Sugar busters! for kids / Samuel S. Andrews . . . [et al.].—1st ed.
p. cm.
Includes bibliographical references and index.
ISBN 0-345-44571-6
1. Carbohydrates, Refined—Pathophysiology. 2. Sugar-free diet. 3. Obesity in
children—Prevention. I. Andrews, Samuel S.
RC627.R43 S843 2001
613.2'83'083—dc21
2001035881

Text design by Holly Johnson

H. Leighton Steward photo © Jackson Hill
All other author photos © Bevil Knapp 5/98

Manufactured in the United States of America

First Edition: August 2001

10 9 8 7 6 5 4 3 2 1

This book is dedicated to all children and the caregivers who endeavor to provide them with a healthy way of life.

A portion of the royalties from each book will be donated to Save the Children®, an organization that has provided assistance to children in need throughout the world since 1932.

Contents

Contents

Part II: Shopping, Cooking, and Eating Sugar Busters Style

Part III: Rhymes for Kids

Acknowledgments

We sincerely appreciate the encouragement of our editor, Maureen O'Neal, and our publisher, Gina Centrello, who have been tremendously supportive in the promotion of this book and our three previous books. Our heartfelt thanks to Walt Handelsman, who with talent and great humor gave vision to Sugar Busters concepts, creating illustrations that are worth more than ten thousand words.

We are grateful for those who have pioneered and are researching the glycemic index concept: David Jenkins, M.D.; Thomas Wolever, M.D.; David Ludwig, M.D.; and Michel Montignac. We acknowledge the dedication of Gerald Berenson, M.D., and other researchers who diligently work in the fields of disease prevention and community health education. We also thank our many other colleagues in the health professions: physicians, nurses, and dietitians who are promoting the Sugar Busters concept as an effective lifestyle for the prevention and remediation of obesity. In particular, we are grateful to Rachel Bollinger, M.S., R.D., Pediatric Dietitian, University of Virginia Medical Center, for her recommendations regarding the specific nutritional needs of children and the development and analysis of this book's meal plans.

We appreciate the commitment of our Web master, Max Maxwell, and our faithful "Sweet Talk" Web site followers for participating in

Acknowledgments

our research survey, promoting the Sugar Busters way of eating, and supporting newcomers in the Sugar Busters lifestyle.

Our gratitude and appreciation go to Linda Andrews and Rita Lapara for their significant contribution to the creation and testing of recipes. We also deeply appreciate the ever-constant, loyal support and enthusiastic encouragement of our families, friends, and followers.

Foreword

I am extremely pleased that the authors of *Sugar Busters! for Kids* have asked me to write a foreword for their book. I accepted at once for two reasons. One, I like to eat, and two (and much more importantly), a proper diet for children is extremely important for their good health. This foreword gives me a wonderful opportunity to emphasize the importance of nutrition and the composition of the diet of children. This book is devoted not only to improving the nutrition of children but also to helping parents become involved with their children in planning and preparing food. For simplicity's sake I will use the generic term *diet*; but this is not a diet book. It is designed to help families and children master healthy foods and good eating habits.

The highly successful book *Sugar Busters! Cut Sugar to Trim Fat* demonstrates how effective the right diet is for adults. Now the authors are focusing on where all good habits should begin—with children. They have adapted recipes to meet the crucial needs of a child's diet.

Our research in the Bogalusa Heart Study has conclusively found that diet is a major factor in raising healthy children. Adult heart disease, heart attacks, strokes, high blood pressure, and diabetes, as well as other chronic health problems, actually begin in childhood. It is critical to understand that habits such as eating behaviors, food choices, and good nutrition also begin in childhood. It is far easier to learn good habits early than to make changes later. In the Bogalusa Heart Study we examined poor diets and poor lifestyles (i.e. smoking, physical inactivity, and accelerating obesity) and from that we developed Health Ahead/Heart Smart, a health education program for elementary school children. We learned that healthy lifestyles can be taught to children even in the face of peer pressure, TV advertising, and other media, and that the impact of this teaching extends to their teachers and parents.

It is encouraging to see people making an effort to improve the nutrition of young children and providing guidance for good menu planning. We have long advocated a balanced diet for growing children. Such a diet consists of adequate *calories* for growth, but not so many that the caloric intake exceeds the child's energy expenditure, which can result in obesity. A mere forty to fifty calorie excess per day (less than one slice of bread or one soft drink) can result in gaining five pounds of extra weight in a year.

An adequate intake of good quality *protein*, including all of the essential amino acids, is needed for growth, regeneration and repair of tissue, and good immunologic health.

Vitamins, minerals, and even *fat* are basic components of a healthy diet. Certain fatty acids, such as the essential acids of poly- and mono-unsaturated fat, are necessary for health. The major culprit leading to adult coronary artery disease is saturated fat. Red meat has received a bad rap because it is a vehicle for saturated fat. Yet lean meat and egg whites contain the most balanced proteins. The optimum amount of vitamins and trace minerals are still under study. For example, optimum levels of vitamin C, vitamin E, and minerals like selenium and zinc are not yet known.

Obesity is dramatically increasing in children. Obesity translates into increased incidence of adult onset Type 2 diabetes, which is now beginning to appear in children. This book is based on the reduction of refined sugar, which is a major contributor to obesity. A burst of sugar in the blood stimulates an excess secretion of insulin and promotes obesity. The Bogalusa Heart Study documented that children today are twelve pounds heavier (but not taller) than their peers were in 1973. We've also demonstrated that over one-third of the offspring of parents with diabetes showed evidence indicating that they will become diabetic as young adults.

Genetics also plays a role in obesity and blood cholesterol levels related to heart disease. But what we really observe is the interaction between genetics and environment. Diet is a major environmental contributor to this interaction. We see too many obese parents, and they often have obese offspring. So take heed of early prevention and pay more attention to the quality of food your children eat. We encourage parents and anyone concerned about the health of children to read this book and improve the dietary behavior of children by involving them in healthy cooking and eating. Planning menus and then helping with cooking make wonderful activities for children.

New ideas and advances will emerge in the future to help refine our diets. Although the emphasis is on avoiding sugar and choosing foods that have a low glycemic index, the authors encourage a diet that meets the general guidelines of the American Heart Association. They stress the need for prevention of obesity through both diet and exercise. Importantly, they encourage children to become interested in their own health. These are general principles that will last a lifetime and help prevent future heart disease. As a physician and preventive cardiologist, I highly recommend this book to parents and children. Childhood is where lifelong healthy habits should begin. The food we eat can be made enjoyable and still be healthy. We have learned a lot since the early 1970s when heart disease was responsible for well over half the deaths in the United States. Changing our diet over the past three decades has contributed to the dramatic decline in heart disease in the adult population and to a much longer life span. Undoubtedly we will learn even more in the future. In the meantime, paying attention to what our children eat and understanding the role of a proper diet sets the stage for what we wish to achieve in preventative medicine. The authors are to be commended for providing this direction.

I wish you good health.

Gerald S. Berenson, M.D.
Distinguished Boyd Professor,
Louisiana State University
Director, Tulane Center for Cardiovascular Health
The Bogalusa Heart Study

Part I

What Is Sugar Busters?

1

Introduction

What if there were a way of eating that included successful weight loss and maintenance of that weight loss? What if that way of eating could be followed without compromising nutritional needs or causing frequent episodes of hunger? What if family members could adopt that way of eating whether they were overweight, of average weight, or underweight? What if that way of eating could decrease risk factors of heart disease, hypertension, and diabetes? What if that way of eating were a plan for living as well as a way of eating? What if that plan had been experienced by millions of individuals and found to be successful? And what if whole families achieved success with that lifestyle? The Sugar Busters lifestyle offers all of this and more, as a solution to families who are concerned about the alarming obesity epidemic and resultant health risks.

With over 2 million copies in print and translations into nineteen languages, we think that *Sugar Busters! Cut Sugar to Trim Fat* is helping to change the way the world eats. We believe the Sugar Busters lifestyle is successful because it is easy to follow and because it is logical, practical, and reasonable. Most diets are diets of exclusion. Sugar Busters offers a lifestyle of healthy choices, inclusion of all food groups, and selection of natural foods with less refined sugar. This way of eating consists of foods that are similar to the unprocessed foods of our ancestors. Few of our ancestors were overweight; only in recent generations have we experienced such widespread obesity.

We are introducing *Sugar Busters! for Kids* because children who learn correct eating habits early in life will not have to struggle with obesity problems later in life. They will not have to face problems with poor self-esteem and the serious risk factors for disease that are complications of obesity. The *Sugar Busters! for Kids* lifestyle offers an easy, straightforward way for parents to help their children learn to make correct food choices and attain lifelong healthy eating habits.

Sugar Busters! for Kids is a wake-up call to rally around the important issue of childhood nutrition and obesity. As conscientious parents, we monitor our children's behavior, study habits, and social interactions. But something has gone very wrong with our attention to our children's nutrition. As a nation, we are not monitoring our children's nourishment and we are not providing the right food choices. This is verified in research, statistics on childhood obesity, and in the increase of diseases related to obesity.

Now over one-half of the adult population of the United States is overweight. In the past decade the incidence of childhood obesity has doubled. Since many adults became overweight as children and have remained that way all of their lives, prevention and early treatment are the best solutions to the obesity epidemic.

What is causing this explosion of weight gain in our children? You have heard the many reasons for the cause of this huge epidemic: less exercise, more inactivity, snacking in front of the TV, the enticement of junk food advertisements, and hurried, working parents' increasing reliance on fast food. All of these issues certainly factor into the cause. However, in our opinion, poor diet is the main reason for the increasing girth of our kids. The tremendous success of the Sugar Busters way of eating, our concerns about increasing obesity as an epidemic for people of all ages, as well as the many requests we have received from followers, have prompted us to develop a Sugar Busters lifestyle for kids.

Sugar Busters! for Kids is written specifically for children. The nutritional and lifestyle concepts presented in our first book, *Sugar*

Busters! Cut Sugar to Trim Fat, are the basis for this new book. However, certain modifications have been made to address the special requirements of our growing kids. Children are *not* small adults. They have their own nutritional demands that must be met to accommodate their ever-changing bodies. *Sugar Busters! for Kids* has been created to accomplish this as well as to incorporate the healthy, nutritional benefits of the Sugar Busters concept into a lifelong plan for healthy eating. Children age two and under should get about half their daily calories from fat for growth and brain development. Therefore, the macronutrient content that we recommend in the daily meal plan is not designed for children age two and under.

This Is Not a Diet Book

Many parents are naturally concerned about putting their children on diets. Diets are hard to follow, hard to stay with, and difficult for parents to monitor. *Sugar Busters! for Kids* is not a diet book. It is not a fad or a quick solution. The word *diet* can mean an individual's *usual* food and drink, or it can refer to a *regulated* selection of foods. Most people think negative thoughts when they hear the word *diet*. We think that families will make Sugar Busters their usual way of eating because it is a positive approach to a healthy lifestyle. We are as interested in a good lifestyle for all children as we are in developing a plan for weight reduction in overweight children.

Heart disease, hypertension, and diabetes are common, chronic, and life-threatening diseases that are associated with obesity. There is increasing evidence that these diseases originate early in life and can be prevented by a proper nutritional lifestyle. *Sugar Busters! for Kids* is not a diet book. Rather, it is a plan for a healthy and nutritious lifestyle with emphasis on disease prevention and favorable weight control.

The Sugar Busters concept is based on control of sugar and insulin. This concept is the foundation of the Sugar Busters lifestyle. We know that high blood sugar (glucose) levels cause high insulin levels that, in turn, may lead to obesity and the diseases associated with obesity.

Sugar Busters is a way of eating that minimizes the elevation of blood sugars and insulin levels. The glycemic index is a measurement of how carbohydrates raise blood sugar and insulin levels. Sugar Busters utilizes the glycemic index as a tool that enables you to recognize how different foods affect your metabolism. Understanding how to use the glycemic index will enable you to make the correct carbohydrate choices.

The Sugar Busters for Kids Lifestyle Includes

1. Reduction of the intake of refined sugar
2. Choice of the correct carbohydrates: consumption of low- or moderate-glycemic carbohydrates instead of high-glycemic carbohydrates
3. Consumption of unprocessed and less processed foods instead of highly processed foods
4. Consumption of whole grains and high-fiber foods
5. Consumption of 30% total fat with fewer than 10% of total calories from saturated fat
6. Regular exercise
7. Limited TV watching, video and computer games
8. Minimal consumption of fast foods
9. Parents as role models

Sugar Busters for Kids will give parents a plan of action for the prevention of childhood obesity while identifying targets for unhealthy eating habits. It will give you a map to chart your course and a rationale for the Sugar Busters lifestyle. You will learn how and why to cut down on refined sugar and also what is lacking in the diets of most children. Since the publication of *Sugar Busters! Cut Sugar to Trim Fat* in 1995, there has been additional research and attention given to the glycemic index, fiber, and whole grains and their impact on weight, health, and longevity. We will review this new and important data and offer suggestions on how you can incorporate this information into your own family's way of eating. A summary of the results of a research survey that we posted on our Web site will inform you of other families' concerns about nutrition and their success with the Sugar Busters lifestyle. We also will identify the foods that overweight children are consuming. A behavior-modification chart, helpful hints, and references will help reinforce your efforts to win an important battle that can determine your child's future health and self-image. You will be given guidelines to determine if your child is overweight. Then you will be provided with meal plans and recipes—some quick and easy that children can prepare themselves, and others that are more detailed. Our "How to Shop and Cook Sugar Busters Style" section will be informative for both newcomers and avid followers. The chapter will be a helpful tool in implementing the Sugar Busters lifestyle. We have met or heard from many of our Sugar Busters followers and will answer the most frequently asked questions. More important, your children can learn about Sugar Busters in a section designed to instruct them in this healthy way of eating. So, whether you are a parent, a child, a new or soon to be Sugar Buster, or a Sugar Busters follower, this book has many new ideas for you.

2

Global Gaining: A Worldwide Epidemic of Obesity in Children

From Beijing to Budapest, Helsinki to Barcelona, and from Boston to San Diego, scientists are investigating the phenomenon of increasing obesity in children. Researchers around the world are finding that childhood obesity is increasing in their countries and should be addressed as a major health concern. Historically obesity has been viewed as a cosmetic problem rather than a health issue. Dieting has been a societal focus for many years for aesthetic reasons. However, now that researchers throughout the world are demonstrating the shocking increase in the incidence of obesity, the serious health consequences have become the primary concern. Parents must be aware that while infectious diseases were the worldwide health epidemics of previous centuries, obesity and diabetes will be the epidemics of the twenty-first century. Could it be that our Western diet is responsible for this global epidemic?

International Studies

A study of over 200,000 children in eleven cities in China concluded that there was a 9% increase in the prevalence of obesity in preschool children each year during the years 1986 to 1996 (Ding). In Europe, more than half of adults are either overweight or obese. These statistics are beginning to correspond to the 55% incidence of overweight individuals in the United States. Researchers are concluding that the problem of obesity is also increasing rapidly among European children and adolescents at an average annual rate of 10%. The prevalence of overweight and obese adolescents in southern Europe is 15% to 25%, which is slightly lower than in the United States (Cruz). As a result, health professionals in Europe are stressing prevention strategies that focus on nutritional education and physical education programs (Martinez).

Several studies evaluated the dietary habits of adolescents in cities in Portugal, Spain, Italy, and Greece. In Catalonia, Spain, the intake of added sugars was very high: 179 grams (45 teaspoons) per day for adolescent males and 107 (27 teaspoons) for adolescent females. A study of schoolchildren in Italy in 1995 indicated that added sugar consumption was 70 grams per day, mostly in the form of white sugar and soft drinks. The surveys in all of the cities studied concluded that large amounts of foods high in sugar and/or fat are being eaten between and during meals. Added sugar accounted for more than 10% of the caloric intake in several studies in southern European countries.

The serum cholesterol levels of adolescents in Spain, Greece, and Italy have increased in the last two decades and are now similar to cholesterol levels in the United States. Research surveys revealed that adolescents in southern Europe are consuming foods high in sugar such as pastries, cakes, and biscuits. They also are consuming foods high in saturated fats, such as meat and dairy products (Cruz). Regrettably, the problem in the United States is more serious because children here are consuming 16% to 20% of their calories from added sugar (Guthrie). These empty sugar calories have no nutritional value and only add to children's weight problems.

The increase in worldwide obesity parallels the increase in sugar consumption. Consumption of excessive fat has been the prime suspect as the cause of heart disease and increasing incidence of obesity. However, even though more and more people have adopted a low-fat diet, obesity is becoming more prevalent. Manufacturers, who are producing foods that are low fat, or fat free, are loading them up with sugar. As any good Sugar Buster knows, most people convert excess sugar and high-glycemic carbohydrates into stored fat. Unfortunately, dieters frequently consume low-fat foods that are high in sugar. For too long, sugar and foods that convert into sugar in the body have been ignored as the prime factor in causing obesity.

Incidence of Childhood Obesity

The Sugar Busters concept has developed a phenomenal worldwide reputation. Now we wish to focus on our country's most valuable resource, our children. Since obesity in children is a major health challenge, *Sugar Busters! for Kids* is devoted to meeting the challenge by calling attention to the crisis and offering a logical plan for intervention and prevention. How is obesity impacting children in the United States?

The incidence of children who are obese and overweight today in the United States has never been higher. Obesity is a measurement of body fat. More than 90% of obese and overweight children have primary obesity, which means they eat too much of the wrong foods. The remaining obese and overweight children have secondary obesity. These secondary causes are uncommon and are due to specific medical disorders such as hypothyroidism, Cushing's syndrome, or Prader-Willi syndrome. Since improper nutrition may not be the only reason for a child's overweight condition, a pediatrician should be consulted to eliminate possible medical causes.

Over the last two decades, childhood obesity has increased at the same rate as obesity in adults. During the 1960s and 1970s in the United States, approximately 5% of children were overweight. Today, 25% of all children and adolescents are overweight or obese. One-third of all infants, 6% to 15% of schoolchildren, and 35% of college students are overweight or obese (Lowry). Unfortunately, most obese adolescents will become obese adults.

Parental factors, both genetic and environmental, play an important role in determining obesity in children. If both parents are obese, there is subsequently an 80% chance of their children being obese. If one parent is obese, there is a 40% chance of their children being obese, and if neither parent is obese, there is only a 15% chance of their children being obese (Attwood). These statistics highlight the importance of parents setting correct nutritional examples for their children. Although some children may inherit a predisposition to obesity from their parents, we believe that parental influence on children's nutrition and physical activity are significant factors in determining whether or not the child will develop obesity. Parents buy the food and plan the menus, so they should be constantly aware that they are both models and guides for their children in making the correct nutritional choices.

Another concern regarding the obesity dilemma is that we as a society are ignoring and denying the repercussions of the problem. Could it be that so many are gaining so much that what once appeared to be overweight is now considered to be a normal weight? A recent study explores this phenomenon. A national survey of over 10,000 men and women in Melbourne, Australia, revealed that many of those who were, in fact, clinically overweight did not identify themselves as such. Fifty percent of the men and 28% of the women who were clinically overweight did not consider themselves to be overweight (Donath). As so many of us become overweight, our perception of what is normal weight can become flawed. Obviously, getting heavier together will not solve the problem. It is time for a realistic approach that includes a way of eating that has been proven to be effective.

The complications of obesity in children are numerous and involve many medical disorders, low self-esteem, depression, and rejection by peers. Obesity-related diseases are becoming more prevalent among our children. Abnormal blood tests are being observed in overweight children, predicting future onset of cardiovascular and metabolic diseases.

Diabetes

One of the most serious consequences of obesity is diabetes mellitus, which is a disorder of carbohydrate metabolism. It is the most common metabolic disease in the world, currently affecting 150 million people. This number is projected to double in twenty-five years. During the past decade, the prevalence of diabetes has increased in the United States by 33%, corresponding to the rapid increase in obesity. Diabetes is the leading cause of kidney failure, loss of a lower extremity, and new cases of adult blindness (Centers for Disease Control). Diabetes more than doubles the risk of heart attack and stroke. This disease has the potential for being seriously incapacitating. Adopting Sugar Busters as a lifestyle may prevent the type of diabetes associated with obesity. Physicians are finding that when they prescribe the Sugar Busters lifestyle for their diabetic patients, their blood sugars are easier to control and the need for insulin and other medications is decreased. This low-glycemic way of eating differs greatly from the typical high-glycemic American diet.

The majority of people with diabetes have either Type 1 diabetes or Type 2 diabetes. These are two distinct and different diseases, although the complications are very similar. There are also less common types of diabetes that can occur during pregnancy (gestational diabetes), the stress associated with a major illness, or during treatment with certain medications.

Type 1 diabetes usually occurs in children and young adults and is characterized by marked insulin deficiency. It typically comes on rapidly, causing a severe metabolic derangement (life-threatening changes in acid-base balance, kidney malfunction, very high blood sugars, and abnormally high blood lipids). Immediate treatment with insulin, intravenous fluids, and electrolytes is required. Once stabilized, the individual will require lifelong daily insulin therapy, diet, and exercise to control the disorder.

Type 2 diabetes is a more insidious and slowly developing disorder, which is characterized by resistance to insulin. Ninety-five percent of all diabetics have Type 2 diabetes. Currently there are 16 million people in the United States with diabetes and that number will double in 15 years, a more rapid rate than the projection for the rest of the world. Type 2 diabetes is becoming so common that almost one million new cases are being diagnosed in this country each year. People who have Type 2 diabetes are not usually insulin deficient, but they are insulin resistant. This means their insulin is not totally effective in lowering blood sugar. Type 2 diabetes, which is typically seen in adults over the age of thirty, can go undiagnosed for many years because of few, if any, specific symptoms. The treatment consists of diet, exercise, oral diabetic medications, and specific treatment for commonly associated problems of hypertension and lipid disorders. Insulin is rarely required during the initial twenty years of the disease.

Prior to 1990, very few children with diabetes had Type 2 diabetes. The number of children with Type 2 diabetes has increased significantly parallelling the increasing rate of obesity among children. Today as many as 30% of newly diagnosed diabetic children have Type 2 diabetes. Before 1990 this disorder was rarely seen in people younger than age forty. However, this disease has been recently diagnosed in a four-year-old child.

Obesity is the most important risk factor for the development of Type 2 diabetes. This means as weight increases above the normal ideal body weight, the chance of developing diabetes increases; and the higher the weight above normal, the greater the incidence of diabetes. Not only are more and more overweight children developing Type 2 diabetes, but also those overweight children who do not develop it as children are at greater risk for developing it as adults. Parents should be aware that if there is a family history of Type 2 diabetes, their children, if overweight, are at a much greater risk for developing this disorder.

Examination of one American population in particular, the Pima Indians who live in the Southwest United States, illustrates how the Western diet has affected the increase in diabetes in one group of people. The typical Western diet consists of high-glycemic carbohydrates and low-fiber foods consumed by much of the population of the Western world. Many scientific papers have been written about the high incidence of diabetes in the Pima Indians. Of all world populations, they now have the highest incidence of this disorder. Over 70% of female Pima Indians, fifty years of age and older, have Type 2 diabetes.

An interesting long-term dietary study of 170 Pima Indians was published in the May 2000 abstracts of the Scientific Sessions of the American Diabetes Association. The long-term effect of diet was correlated with the development of Type 2 diabetes in the Indian population. The Pima Indians studied followed three kinds of diets. The first group consumed a traditional Pima Indian diet consisting of desert foods, pinto beans, other legumes, and high-fiber vegetables. The second group consumed a typical Western or Anglo diet of meat, bread, and potatoes. The third group consumed a mixed diet consisting of foods in both the traditional Indian diet and the Western diet. The rate of diabetes in the Western or Anglo diet group was 5 times higher than in the traditional Pima Indian diet group. The rate of diabetes in the mixed diet group was 2.3 times higher than the traditional Pima Indian diet group. The researchers concluded that eating a Western-style diet often leads to the development of diabetes in Pima Indians (Williams). This dramatic increase in diabetes in the Pima Indian population illustrates the hazards of the Western diet. It is obvious that the worldwide epidemic of diabetes is due more to unhealthy diet than to genetics. If an individual has a genetic predisposition to diabetes, eating foods that elevate blood sugars and insulin levels increases the risk for development of the disease. Obesity and consumption of a Western-style diet are responsible for the enormous numbers of people developing Type 2 diabetes and will continue to fuel the epidemic.

Heart Disease

A startling fact is that risk factors for heart disease are also occurring in overweight children and adolescents. Although much recent attention has been focused on findings that the initial stages of heart disease develop in childhood, this is not a new area of investigation. Dr. Gerald Berenson, the director of the Bogalusa Heart Study, has written over 700 scientific articles on this subject. Dr. Berenson and other scientists studied 16,000 children for thirty years as they grew up in the small town of Bogalusa in southeast Louisiana. The project was developed to detect early signs of heart disease in children. Results of this research revealed that the seeds for heart disease begin early in life and are related to the unhealthy conditions of obesity, lack of exercise, and smoking. The investigators found elevated cholesterol levels, high blood pressure, and high insulin levels in grade-school children (Berenson). Dr. Berenson has demonstrated that prevention and treatment of obesity in childhood has the potential to reduce the risk of heart disease in adulthood (Freedman).

Not only has the Bogalusa Heart Study identified elevated insulin levels in young children, but the study also has shown that these elevated levels persist into young adulthood, resulting in increased risk for heart disease. High insulin levels occur in obese children and also can occur in children destined to become obese. Elevated insulin levels are known to be independent risk factors for the development of heart disease and Type 2 diabetes.

Other Conditions

Moderate to severe asthma is more prevalent in overweight children. Obesity is also the most important risk factor for pediatric hypertension (high blood pressure). Orthopedic problems, such as hip and lower extremity deformities with associated pain and decreased range of motion, are more frequent among obese children. Psychological effects, such as low self-esteem, depression, eating disorders, and the stigma that leads to rejection by peers, are much more frequent among obese children. Sleep apnea can occur in obese children and is believed to contribute to learning difficulties and failure in school.

Abnormal growth acceleration is seen in obese children, with females often demonstrating premature puberty. Lipid (fat) abnormalities in the blood are often detected in cholesterol screenings of obese children. These abnormalities include increased triglycerides, increased total cholesterol, increased LDL (bad) cholesterol, and decreased HDL (good) cholesterol. This biochemical pattern is certainly atherogenic (produces hardening of the arteries) in adults and puts these children at an increased risk of developing advanced arteriosclerosis when they reach adulthood. As adults, they also would be in jeopardy of having strokes and heart attacks at an earlier age.

All of the complications of obesity are commonly seen in medical practice, and the consequences are serious both for quality of life and longevity. A Harvard study that began in 1922 showed that adolescent obesity was associated with increased risk of mortality in all disorders studied, particularly coronary artery disease and colon cancer. Being overweight in adolescence was a much more significant predictor of disease than being overweight in adulthood (Must). Medical research continues to document the devastating effects of childhood and adolescent obesity.

Western Diet

Almost everyone agrees that more long-term research is needed to determine specific and effective nutritional guidelines for children. But because too many children are at risk, we believe that intervention must come before the results of long-term studies are available. We must use the research that is currently available to arrive at a logical and reasonable nutritional plan. *Sugar Busters! for Kids* is that plan. Without exception, hundreds of studies conclude that the obesity crisis will not resolve without intervention. Unfortunately, most of the research projects focus on identifying the problem without suggesting a specific cause or remedy. We are concerned with the lack of consensus on how to target the problem.

Most health professionals and researchers have concluded that improved nutrition and increased physical exercise are necessary to prevent and remedy obesity. However, current nutritional guidelines do not seem to be effecting any positive change. Most experts have suggested a significant decrease in fat consumption as a solution to the problem. Data from the Third National Health and Nutrition Examination Survey (NHANES III) indicate that although total fat and saturated fat intake in our population has decreased since the 1960s, the obesity epidemic is increasing. Reduced fat and reduced caloric intake from the use of low-calorie food products have been associated with a paradoxical increase in the rate of obesity (Heini).

Sugar consumption is soaring; foods are becoming more processed; TV watching, computer use, and video-game playing are increasing. The golden arches of fast-food restaurants are stretching globally. Parents must be able to recognize a present or potential weight problem in their children and have both the plan and the determination to effect a change.

Our Western diet consists of a high intake of refined sugar and highly processed carbohydrates, and a low intake of fruits, vegetables, and whole grains. Typical fast-food fare also has become the hallmark of this diet. We think that the Western diet and the increased Westernization of diets throughout the world is the major contributor to the obesity problem.

The negative aspects of the Western diet are demonstrated in a 1997 study of 13,783 adolescents. The survey showed that second-generation children of immigrants in this country are significantly more overweight than their parents. Thirty-one percent of second-generation Asian immigrant groups, except Chinese and Filipinos, were overweight compared to 15.6% of first-generation Asian Americans. This indicates a doubling of the number of overweight individuals between the first and second generations. The Hispanic children of immigrants also showed a significant increase in the number of overweight children between generations (Popkin). Since this problem occurred with immigration to this country, the phenomenon appears to be nutritional and environmental, rather than genetic. We conclude from the data in the immigrant study that the Westernized diet and lifestyle have a significantly greater influence in determining obesity than heredity.

Few will argue that the quality of life in our great country is high. There is much prosperity. We are exporting great products, ideas, and technologies. However, we are exporting one concept that needs changing: the Western diet of refined sugar, overprocessed grains, and fast foods. We are exporting too much of the sweet life, and the sweet life is leading to a global epidemic.

3

The Sugar Busters Concept

We hope that we have convinced you of the gravity and pervasiveness of the obesity crisis, because identifying the problem is the first step in determining a solution. Every day we hear from more and more families who have adopted the Sugar Busters lifestyle. These families are discovering that the Sugar Busters way of eating is a successful plan for the entire family. We will tell you more about the good results when we discuss the very informative data from the questionnaires answered by parents. Because Sugar Busters is really a family affair, we want to first familiarize you with the basic Sugar Busters concept before we offer specific guidelines for your children.

Sugar Busters is a nutritional lifestyle, not just another fad diet. It is about how, what, and when to eat. Yes, it does involve exercise. You will find that Sugar Busters is logical, practical, and reasonable, and you will not be burdened by having to weigh, count, and measure foods. Because we encourage you to avoid refined sugar and processed grain products, Sugar Busters will be a "less-sugar" diet than most of you are probably following, but it is definitely not a "no-sugar" diet. In fact, we strongly encourage you to make a commitment to choosing correct carbohydrates that are the low-insulin-producing carbohydrates, which are necessary for the proper function of your body. Insulin causes the body to convert and store excess carbohydrates (sugar) as fat, and can lead to obesity. You cannot live *without* insulin, but you can live much better without *too much* insulin. By choosing correct carbohydrates such as those in whole-grain and high-fiber foods, you will lessen the insulin requirements and reduce the peaks and valleys of insulin you experience throughout the day. According to Guyton and Hall's most recent textbook of medical physiology, excess carbohydrates not used immediately for energy or stored in the glycogen deposits (in liver and muscle) are converted to fat and stored as such.

The Sugar Busters way of eating involves consumption of high-fiber vegetables, fruits, and whole grains. The fiber in these foods has a beneficial effect on your digestive process and overall health. Eating fruits is encouraged in the Sugar Busters lifestyle; fruit makes an excellent snack. Meat is an important source of protein, but any meat eaten should be lean and trimmed of fat before cooking. Sugar Busters is cautious about fat—especially saturated fat. We recommend that when selecting milk and cheese products, you choose those with a reduced fat content. We strongly advocate limiting saturated fats. Too much saturated fat and trans-fats (oils used in fast foods) are very harmful—not only to your waistline, but also to your heart and blood vessels. Hydration is important, and everyone is encouraged to drink six to eight glasses of water daily. Skipping meals is not healthy. It is important to eat three regular meals daily, as well as appropriate snacks. But moderation in portion size is most important. If you are not careful, you can easily eat too much of even a correct food choice. Late-night snacking is not allowed. Eating before going to bed only raises your insulin level and encourages cholesterol production, since most cholesterol is manufactured while you are sleeping.

Exercise is an important part of any successful nutritional lifestyle. You should strive to exercise vigorously at least twenty to thirty minutes, four days per week to raise your heart rate. However, some people may be overambitious about exercise, and when they do not meet their expectations they just give up. They bite off more (exercise) than they can chew (perform). A little exercise will go a long way and certainly is better than none at all.

Sugar Busters is *selective* rather than *restrictive*. You can choose food from all four food groups, but we encourage you to make the best selections within each food group. Sugar Busters is the voice of moderation since it is a reasonable, not an extreme or radical, approach to nutrition. It has been developed to encourage compliance rather than cheating. Sugar Busters is a great plan that is easy to follow, and the closer you follow it the better your results.

4

The Glycemic Index

The glycemic index is the main tool of the Sugar Busters lifestyle. Understanding this concept is basic to understanding why Sugar Busters works. Before you decide to skip this chapter, which may sound too technical, give us a chance to explain in simple terms how to become an astute Sugar Busters scientist.

If you log onto the chat room on our Web site (*www.sugarbusters.com*) or attend one of the authors' presentations, you will be impressed with the depth of understanding that followers of the Sugar Busters concept have developed. We believe that individuals need to know and understand the scientific explanation for this concept. Our followers have done their homework. They not only know that the Sugar Busters lifestyle is successful for them, but also why the Sugar Busters lifestyle works. It is easy to follow a plan that is logical, practical, and reasonable, and that provides excellent results.

The glycemic index is a measure of how carbohydrates differ in their ability to elevate blood sugars and insulin levels after they are digested. Carbohydrates are not created equally. The physical properties of carbohydrates cause them to be digested at different rates. The more rapidly digested carbohydrates produce the greatest rise in blood sugar. These carbohydrates are known as high-glycemic carbohydrates. Some carbohydrates digest more slowly, and these are called moderate- or low-glycemic carbohydrates. When carbohydrates, such as whole grains, have outer layers of bran, the digestive enzymes are delayed in doing their job. This slows down the digestion of these foods. Consuming fiber, fat, and protein with carbohydrates can also slow down the digestion of carbohydrates. All of these processes lower blood-sugar levels. Remember, this is what we are attempting to achieve: slower digestion of carbohydrates, lower blood-sugar levels, lower insulin levels, and less fat storage. We can accomplish this by the consumption of low-glycemic carbohydrates. Our reward: normal weight and better health!

The glycemic index is also an indicator of how different carbohydrates react in the body. Carbohydrates are either simple or complex. Simple carbohydrates are sugars: for example, table sugar or candy. Complex carbohydrates are basically grains, legumes, and starches such as potatoes.

The complex carbohydrates are composed of many glucose molecules attached to one another. After the complex carbohydrates are eaten, the digestive enzymes act by breaking the bonds holding the glucose molecules together. The glucose is then taken into the bloodstream. The blood glucose (sugar) begins to rise, and this increase in blood sugar stimulates the pancreas to release insulin to match the elevated level of blood sugar. Low-glycemic carbohydrates cause a low level of insulin secretion. This is the reason Sugar Busters encourages consumption of low-glycemic carbohydrates rather than high-glycemic carbohydrates.

Glucose acts both as a fuel to be utilized immediately and as a future source of energy. Glucose first replaces the glycogen in muscles and the liver that has been depleted overnight or after vigorous exercise. Glycogen serves as an energy source for the release of glucose during overnight fasting. After the glycogen has been replenished by the glucose, any excess is converted into fat. The fat is then stored as triglycerides, especially in the abdominal area.

This process of carbohydrates or glucose converting into fat is called *de novo lipogenesis*. This is a phenomenon that occurs in certain animals that eat excessive amounts of carbohydrates and store them as fat. These animals, such as bears, eat large amounts of carbohydrates in the summer and fall, storing them as fat for the winter hibernation. However, if humans eat this way, since humans don't hibernate, any stored fat is usually still there in the spring. In fact, the average American gains several pounds from Thanksgiving until January 2 because of all of the sweets and other high-glycemic carbohydrates eaten during the holidays. This holiday-induced weight gain tends to stay with us and leads to girth instead of mirth!

We know that certain carbohydrates more easily raise the blood sugar and insulin to high levels, causing the body to convert excess carbohydrates into fat. The premise of Sugar Busters is that the consumption of these high-glycemic carbohydrates causes excessive insulin secretion, which leads to obesity and other diseases. A diet that consists of high-glycemic carbohydrates leads to the conversion of glucose (sugar) into fat. High insulin levels also inhibit the breakdown of the stored fat. This biochemical process will cause an individual to remain in a fat-storage mode, perpetuating obesity. A high insulin level is a double-edged sword; it causes storage of fat and prevents the breakdown of fat.

Dr. David Jenkins of Toronto, Canada, did much of the early work on the glycemic index. He is a professor at the University of Toronto and a physician. The glycemic index is not a new concept. It has been around since Dr. Jenkins's original work in 1981 (Jenkins). The glycemic index has been extensively researched and adopted as a sound nutritional principle in Canada, New Zealand, England, Australia, and India. More recently Italy and Sweden have joined in research on this theory that has changed the way we look at nutrition and carbohydrate metabolism.

The United States has been slow to recognize the importance of the concept that carbohydrates differ in their nutritional effects. As with many new positive and revolutionary ideas and theories, change takes time. Since the publication of our original book, *Sugar Busters! Cut Sugar to Trim Fat*, in 1995, public and professional awareness of the value of the glycemic index has mushroomed. This awareness has become a grassroots movement that has been adopted and promoted by thousands of people. In spite of initial skepticism by some, proponents have endorsed the cause with unrelenting tenacity. Why? Simply because the plan works. It works for the overweight. It works for diabetics. It works for those with elevated cholesterol and other lipid abnormalities. It also works for those with symptoms of digestive acid reflux and hypoglycemia.

Just what are high-glycemic carbohydrates and how do we identify them? Dr. Jenkins originally pioneered work in this area. He and other scientists have devised a method to test carbohydrates and determine their glycemic index (Wolever).

When a specific carbohydrate is tested, 50 grams of glucose are given to several fasting individuals. The subjects' blood sugars are then measured. On another day, 50 grams of the test carbohydrate are given to the same fasting individuals and their blood sugars are measured again. The subjects' blood sugars are plotted on a graph and compared. Glucose is assigned a number of 100 for 100%, and other carbohydrates are compared to this standard. Glucose is usually the standard by which other carbohydrates are classified in the glycemic index. In some studies, white bread has been used as the standard instead of glucose. We prefer that glucose be used as a standard, because the composition of white bread can vary from country to country and cause inconsistent results.

Refer to the graph at the end of this chapter for a comparison of potatoes (a high-glycemic carbohydrate) and lentils (a low-glycemic carbohydrate). You can see how these carbohydrates compare to glucose, which is the standard. This example demonstrates that potatoes, with a glycemic index of 95, when consumed will raise your blood sugar almost as high as glucose. Lentils, with a glycemic index of 29, minimally raise the blood sugar. This illustrates how important it is to compare carbohydrates and then choose correct carbohydrates. Over the years, researchers have tested many carbohydrates so that now we have access to many glycemic indices. The glycemic indices for over 100 foods can be found at the end of this chapter.

An undesirable side effect of eating high-glycemic foods is hypoglycemia (low blood sugar). The elevated insulin levels stimulated by the wrong kind of carbohydrates force the blood sugar levels down. At times the blood sugar may be driven down below normal, causing mild hypoglycemia. The symptoms of hypoglycemia are irritability, anxiety, sweating, tremors, headache, fainting, and hunger. Hypoglycemia can occur several hours after eating a high-glycemic carbohydrate, causing a person to eat more at the next meal. Many people report that the Sugar Busters way of eating has dramatically relieved their symptoms of hypoglycemia.

Since the publication of our original book, there has been research on the effects of the glycemic index in children. Dr. David Ludwig at Children's Hospital in Boston has demonstrated the effects of a low-glycemic carbohydrate breakfast on children. Ludwig found that appetite for the luncheon meal decreased in children who ate low-glycemic carbohydrates for breakfast (Ludwig). We believe that adults and children who consume low-glycemic foods instead of high-glycemic foods feel more satiated. When you substitute a breakfast of oatmeal or high-fiber unsweetened cereal for sugar-coated cereal or donuts, you are not only helping your child feel satisfied until lunch, you are making it easier to limit his or her food intake at the next meal.

We believe that for the millions of successful Sugar Busters the concept is a lifestyle, not a diet. This is true simply because there is no deprivation. Low- or moderate-glycemic foods are substituted for high-glycemic foods. Refined sugar is restricted and eventually will not even be craved or missed by most people.

Glucose G.I.(Standard)
G.I.=100

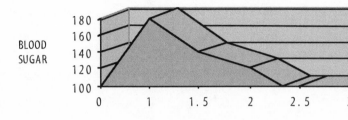

BLOOD SUGAR

180
160
140
120
100

0   1   1.5   2   2.5   3

TIME (HOURS)

Lentil   G.I.(Low)
G.I.=29

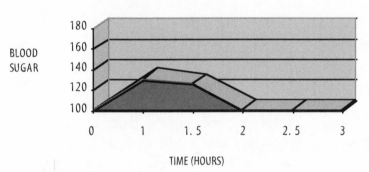

BLOOD SUGAR

180
160
140
120
100

0   1   1.5   2   2.5   3

TIME (HOURS)

White Potato   G.I.(High)
G.I.=95

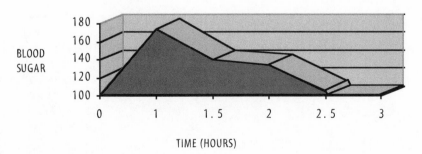

BLOOD SUGAR

180
160
140
120
100

0   1   1.5   2   2.5   3

TIME (HOURS)

5

The Glycemic Index Tables

The medical journal article "International Tables of Glycemic Index" (Foster-Powell) is a listing of hundreds of carbohydrates that have been tested and given values. The glycemic index (GI) values listed below come from that article, except for the Mexican foods (Noriega). If the food was tested more than once, either an average or a range may be used. For practical purposes there is no difference between a glycemic index of 70 and one of 67. There is clearly a difference be- tween a glycemic index of 95 and one of 50. The glycemic indices listed below are all based on the standard glucose, which is assigned a glycemic index of 100.

Breakfast Cereals

All-Bran	42
Corn Chex	83
Corn Flakes	84
Cream of Wheat	66
Cream of Wheat, Instant	74
Crispix	87
Grapenuts	67
Grapenuts Flakes	80
Life	66
Muesli, toasted	43
Muesli, nontoasted	56
Nutri-Grain	66
Oat Bran	55
Oatmeal	55
Puffed Wheat	67
Rice Chex	89
Rice Krispies	82
Shredded Wheat	67
Special K	54

Dairy Products

Chocolate milk, sugar added	34
Milk	27
Milk, skim	32
Yogurt, artificial sweetener	14

Fruits

Apples	36
Apricots, dried	31
Banana (unripe to ripe)	30–70
Cherries	22
Grapefruit	25
Grapefruit juice, unsweetened	48
Grapes	43
Kiwi	52
Mango	55
Orange	43
Orange juice (frozen)	57
Peach	28
Peach, canned, in heavy syrup	58
Pear	36
Pineapple	66
Plum	24
Raisins	64
Watermelon	77

Pasta

Linguine, thin durum	55
Rice pasta	92
Spaghetti, durum boiled 20 min.	64
Spaghetti, white boiled 20 min.	58
Spaghetti, whole wheat	37

Grains and Cereals

Barley	25
Barley, cracked	50
Basmati rice	58
Brown rice	55
Buckwheat	54
Bulgur	48
Corn, sweet	60
Cornmeal	68
Couscous	65
Instant rice	91
Millet	71
Oatmeal	55
Rye, whole	34
Wheat, whole	41
White rice	70–91
Wild rice	57

Soups

Black bean	64
Green pea	66
Lentil	44
Split pea	60
Tomato	38

Beans and Peas

Black beans (Mexican)	30
Brown beans (Mexican)	38
Butter beans	31
Chickpeas	33
Green beans	30
Green peas	48
Kidney beans	27
Lentils	29
Lima beans	32
Navy beans	31
Pinto beans	39
Pinto beans, canned	45
Red beans	26
Soybeans	18
Split peas, yellow	32
Yellow teparies (Pima)	29

Root Vegetables

Beets	64
Carrots	72–112
Baked white potato	94
New potato	62
French fries	75
Sweet potato	54
Yam	51

THE GLYCEMIC INDEX TABLES

Sugars

Fructose	23
Glucose	100
Honey	73
Lactose	46
Maltose	105
Sucrose	75

THE GLYCEMIC INDEX TABLES

37

Mexican Foods

Beans	13
Corn tortilla	52
Corn tortilla bean taco	39
Corn tortilla potato taco	78
Wheat tortilla	30
Wheat tortilla bean taco	28

THE GLYCEMIC INDEX TABLES

6

Whole Grains

Did you ever think that you would tell your children to eat in an unrefined way? Well, that is just what we are advising you to do. The consumption of unrefined whole grains is another important Sugar Busters concept. Whole grains, particularly those that are stone-ground, are recommended instead of processed grains, such as white flour and white rice, because the more the food is processed, the higher its glycemic index. The reason whole grains are so much better nutritionally than refined grains is because whole grains contain higher amounts of fiber, minerals, plant estrogens, and vitamins, especially vitamin E.

Grains can be so refined during the milling process that all of the health benefits are stripped from them. Unprocessed whole grains have their outer layer of bran intact. This layer surrounds the carbohydrate portion of the grain. Like fiber, the outer bran layer of the grain slows down the digestion of a carbohydrate. But when the bran layer is removed, the grain changes from a low-glycemic carbohydrate to a high-glycemic carbohydrate. You have learned the significance of consuming low-glycemic carbohydrates to keep blood sugar and insulin levels low.

Cereal grains make up over 50% of the diet that most populations eat. Since 8500 B.C., man has grown crops of wheat and barley in the

Fertile Crescent of the Near East. Of the twelve major crops grown in the world today, five are cereal grains: wheat, rice, corn, barley, and sorghum (Diamond). Although wheat is the major cereal grain currently consumed, the use of the other grains would be very beneficial because they have a lower glycemic index. Whole barley has a glycemic index of 25, and oat bran has a glycemic index of 55. Compare this to the glycemic index of white flour, which is 70.

The fiber in fruits and vegetables has long been touted for its significance in disease prevention. More recently, whole grains have been found to have health benefits independent of fiber. They contain phytochemicals, antioxidants, and other beneficial nutrients that are not found in fiber. Research is demonstrating that whole grains and fiber work together synergistically (with a potent combined action) to prevent disease.

A lesson in whole grains is a lesson in prevention. It is recommended that children eat at least three servings of whole grains per day. In actuality, many children are not even consuming one serving. Both the nutrients and fiber present in whole grains act to help prevent obesity, heart disease, cancer, and Type 2 diabetes.

Many studies are demonstrating that a wide range of substances in whole grains seem to protect us against several diseases. A 1998 study of over 34,000 women in Iowa indicated that women whose diets consisted of the highest number of servings of whole-grain foods had much lower incidence of death from heart disease (Jacobs). Another study, conducted by the Division of Preventive Medicine of Harvard Medical School, involved a ten-year study of over 65,000 female nurses. This study demonstrated a strong correlation between coronary heart disease and low whole-grain consumption. The researchers concluded that increased intake of whole grains might protect against coronary heart disease (Liu).

Not only do whole grains protect against heart disease, but there is strong evidence that they protect against cancers of the digestive and respiratory tract. A study in Lausanne, Switzerland, involving 500 subjects showed an increase in cancers of the oral cavity, esophagus, pharynx, and larynx in those who consumed refined grains as compared to those who consumed whole grains (Levi). Another study in Milan, Italy, published in 1999 and involving over 5,000 hospitalized patients, demonstrated a significant association between refined grain consumption and cancers of the oral cavity, pharynx, esophagus, larynx, stomach, colon, and thyroid (Chatenoud). Refined grains such as white bread, white pasta, and white rice are high-glycemic carbohydrates that cause high insulin secretion. The high insulin levels may stimulate tumor-cell growth.

If whole grains are so beneficial for us, why is their consumption so low? One of the identified problems is that most people are not familiar with whole grains, how to look for them in the grocery store, or how to prepare them. The most common varieties of grain are wheat, corn, oats, and rice. Breads, cereals, pasta, and crackers are made from grains. Breakfast is a perfect time to eat whole grains because oatmeal and some ready-to-eat cereals are whole-grain foods. And, there are plenty of whole-grain options for lunch and dinner as you will learn in our "How to Shop and Cook Sugar Busters Style" section. Stock your pantry with whole-grain breads, crackers, pastas, and brown rice. Look for barley, bulgur, buckwheat, pumpernickel, couscous, and muesli on grocery shelves and on restaurant menus as alternatives to white potatoes, white bread, and white rice. Be careful to avoid those whole grains that have added refined sugar. In a later chapter you will learn how to avoid highly refined products and foods with added sugars by paying close attention to the ingredients listed on package labels.

Fortunately, ancient grains are being reintroduced into our diet to add health benefits and variety. It is interesting that more and more food magazines and cookbooks are featuring recipes with whole grains. Take advantage of this significant rediscovery and make whole grains a vital part of your family's way of eating.

7

Where Has All the Fiber Gone?

Fiber has inconspicuously and gradually crept out of the diets of developed countries over the last century. At one time our ancestors consumed every plant that was not toxic. Currently, dietary fiber is consumed less in the United States than in any other country in the world. The average United States citizen consumes 12 grams of fiber a day, while people in South American countries consume 25 grams, and people in Mediterranean countries consume 38 grams per day (Spiller). In underdeveloped countries, where dietary fiber is an important component of the daily diet, obesity is rare. In developed and developing countries, where the intake of dietary fiber is lower, the incidence of obesity is rapidly increasing.

For thousands of years our ancestors ate a high-fiber, unprocessed-carbohydrate diet. With the increase of industrialization and urbanization fewer people continued to grow their own grain. Grain was processed at a centralized mill and stored. This necessitated a change in processing because whole grains cannot be preserved for long periods of time without risk of spoilage. The whole-grain kernel contains germ oil that tends to become rancid over time. The solution was to process wheat until it became white flour. That is where the fiber went: onto the mill floor. We sacrificed better nutrition for convenience!

Fiber is either soluble or insoluble in water. Dried beans, oats, barley, and some fruits and vegetables have high levels of soluble fiber. Whole grains, wheat bran, cereals, seeds, and the skins of many fruits and vegetables are foods that are high in insoluble fiber. Insoluble fiber is not digestible, so it provides bulk, which fills the stomach, therefore less food is consumed. It also has few calories. Nutritionists recommend a minimum of 20 to 30 grams of fiber each day. The Sugar Busters program recommends 30 to 35 grams of fiber per day. That is far above the amount that most children are currently consuming, so you have to be inventive, creative, and persistent in your efforts to include foods in your family's diet that are high in fiber. Our daily meal plans and food fiber chart will guide you in increasing this important component of the Sugar Busters lifestyle.

Advantages of High-Fiber Foods

Foods rich in fiber are very filling. The roughage naturally cuts down on the amount of food consumed at each meal. This characteristic of fiber can therefore decrease your appetite and the amount of food you consume at your next meal and also can diminish the amount of snacking that occurs between meals. Another reason that high-fiber foods can decrease your appetite is because they usually have a lower glycemic index. Remember that foods with a low glycemic index stimulate less insulin. When less insulin is secreted, appetite can be decreased. People who consume high-fiber foods also tend to cut down on high-fat and high-sugar foods.

Cholesterol levels are lower in people who eat a high-fiber diet. In addition to consuming fewer high-cholesterol foods, eating fiber inhibits the production of cholesterol in the body. High-fiber diets also reduce the elevation of blood sugar and insulin. High insulin levels are related to obesity and also stimulate cholesterol production by the liver.

In a Harvard study of 65,173 nurses, the incidence of Type 2 diabetes was more than twice as high in nurses who consumed low cereal-fiber breakfasts and a diet with high-glycemic carbohydrates than the nurses who consumed high cereal-fiber breakfasts and low-glycemic carbohydrates. The nurses who developed diabetes consumed large amounts of cola beverages, white bread, white rice, french-fried potatoes, and cooked potatoes. The Harvard researchers recommend that grains should be consumed in a minimally refined form to lessen the development of Type 2 diabetes (Salmeron, Manson). The results were the same in a similar study of 42,759 men (Salmeron, Ascherio).

A diet high in fiber and whole grains, with plenty of water (six to eight glasses per day), is very helpful in the prevention of constipation. This is a condition parents often ask about and which frequently can be remedied with dietary changes. You should also be aware that increases in fiber and whole grains in the diet should be gradual to avoid the occasional mild stomach upset that can occur. The benefits of fiber far outweigh any minor initial side effects.

After considering all of the preventative health advantages of fiber, it becomes clear why it is another major component of the Sugar Busters lifestyle. With all of the known benefits of fiber, we must, paradoxically, move forward by regressing to a more unrefined way of eating. Our ancestors probably were not aware of the importance of fiber. Now that we are, it should be reintroduced as a vital part of our diet.

The sample meals and fiber food tables that follow are guides to assist you in bringing high-fiber foods into your family's diet.

Figure 2: Examples of High-Fiber Meals
(Fiber listed in grams)

Breakfast	Lunch	Dinner
1 slice whole-grain bread (2 g)	2 slices whole wheat bread (4 g)	1 cup red beans (6 g)
1 cup berries (2 g)	1 tablespoon no-sugar-added peanut butter (2 g)	1/2 cup brown rice (2 g)
1/4 cup Kellogg's All-Bran cereal (5 g)	1 apple (2 g)	1/2 cup spinach (2 g)
1/2 cup 1% milk		1 kiwi (3 g)
Subtotal: 9 g	Subtotal: 8 g	Subtotal: 13 g
Total for Day: 30 g		

Figure 3: Fiber Table*

Food Group	Moderate (2g)	High (3g)	Highest (4 g or >)
Breads, Cereals	1 slice whole-grain bread 1 slice rye bread 4 whole wheat crackers 3 Triscuits 1/2 whole-grain pita 1/2 whole-grain bagel		1 cup whole-grain cereal 1/2 cup dry oatmeal or oat bran
Starches	1/2 cup brown rice 1/2 cup whole wheat pasta 1/2 cup shredded wheat	1 sweet potato	
Vegetables	1/2 cup cooked or 1 cup raw asparagus, green beans, broccoli, cabbage, cauliflower, greens, onions, snow peas, spinach, squash, tomatoes, celery, green peppers, or zucchini		
Fruit	1 cup berries 1 apple, nectarine, orange, peach, or plum 1/2 cup grapefruit or pear	1 mango 1 kiwi	
Beans		1/2 cup three-bean salad	1/2 cup cooked lima, black, garbanzo, kidney, or pinto beans, 1/4 cup cooked lentils, 1/2 cup soybeans
Nuts and Seeds	10 almonds, 6 walnuts, or 15 peanuts, 1 tbsp peanut butter, 1 tbsp sesame seeds, 1 tbsp sunflower seeds		

*Use whole-grain unprocessed foods

8

Macronutrients

Macronutrients are proteins, fats, and carbohydrates. They are the nutrients that are required in the greatest amounts in our diets to provide adequate nutrition. Our recommendation of macronutrient composition for children is as follows:

Carbohydrates: 50%; Fat: 30%; Protein: 20%

The macronutrient or major nutrient composition recommended for children in our daily meal plan is based on the Sugar Busters concept and the macronutrients generally recommended by pediatric specialists. *Sugar Busters! for Kids* is not a low-fat diet. It is not a high-protein diet. It is not a high- or low-carbohydrate diet. It is an extremely well-balanced way of eating. The macronutrient composition for adults following Sugar Busters is carbohydrates 40%, fats 30%, and proteins 30%. The close similarity between the two plans permits entire families to benefit from the Sugar Busters lifestyle following easy meal plans.

Let's look at the components of this plan. We recommend that 50% of the diet be carbohydrates. These carbohydrates must be *correct carbohydrates*. This is our term for high-fiber, whole-grain carbohydrates that are not highly processed. People who consume more than a

50% carbohydrate diet are usually overweight. Consuming less than 40% to 50% carbohydrates cuts down on your fiber intake. Consuming less than 20% carbohydrates usually causes both bad breath and ketosis. A severely restricted carbohydrate diet can be unhealthy and very difficult to follow.

We recommend an intake of 30% fat. This is the same amount of total fat that is recommended for adults. The total amount of **saturated** fat should be limited to 10%. In a recent study, researchers compared a high-carbohydrate, low-fat diet (75% carbohydrate, 10% fat) to a diet similar to Sugar Busters (50% carbohydrate, 30% fat). The researchers found that fat synthesis and storage was nine to twenty-seven times higher in the low-fat (10% fat) diet than in the 30% fat diet (Hudgins). This seminal scientific study reinforces the Sugar Busters concept that eating excessive amounts of high-glycemic carbohydrates causes the production and storage of fat and makes weight loss difficult.

Lower fat consumption in children is controversial for several reasons, mainly because as fat decreases in the diet, carbohydrates and simple sugars increase. This dietary change leads to higher blood sugars, higher insulin levels, and more fat storage. This occurs because, in many instances, the fats in commercially prepared foods have been replaced by sugars. Individuals on low-fat diets may also do this, replacing sugar for fat, not realizing that the sugar converts into fat. Diets too low in fat can be detrimental. Research indicates that low-fat diets with 20% or less fat have been associated with growth problems (Dwyer).

The amount of protein that we recommend is 20%. This is well above the minimum needed for growth and development of muscles, yet contains enough amino acids to enable the body to make sugar if needed. It is not so much protein that the kidneys become overwhelmed.

Although macronutrients make up the predominant composition of daily diets, micronutrients are vital. Micronutrients are essential substances that are required in very small amounts in foods but are necessary for nutrition. Iron, vitamins, and calcium are examples of micronutrients. Our meal plan has been designed to exceed the minimum daily requirements for micronutrients.

The Sugar Busters way of eating is much more balanced than many other so-called "healthy diets." Consumption of three meals a day is essential. High fiber at the breakfast meal will not only provide satiety until lunch, but will also cut down on the amount of food consumed at that meal. Snacks are designed to provide much-needed added fiber from fruit, nuts, and vegetables that may not be consumed during meals. While following Sugar Busters you will consume foods from each food group and the proper amounts of both micronutrients and macronutrients.

9

Exercise

There has been a steady decline in physical activity in children over the past decades. Many believe that there is a link between obesity and less physical activity. With the decrease in physical activity, we have seen a rise in the sedentary time in front of the TV and computer, and of course a rise in the weight of children. Exercise was once a vital component of every school curriculum. Now it is all too frequently a minor or nonexistent part of the school day. Recess is being eliminated in many elementary schools throughout the country. The repercussions of this are serious. Safe, supervised school physical education offers an alternative for children who are not able to play outdoors because they reside in high-crime areas. Supervised physical activity in school may be the only opportunity for some children to engage in any vigorous exercise.

The Sugar Busters lifestyle includes regular physical exercise for kids because physical inactivity is also a major risk factor for the development of coronary artery disease and increases the risk of high blood pressure and stroke. Physical inactivity also usually means more time in front of the TV and computer, with more opportunity for snacking. Exercise can lower insulin levels in children who have elevated levels, and it can also improve blood-sugar levels (McMurray). Elevated insulin levels are associated with the development of heart disease and Type 2 diabetes.

Another very important reason why we stress the need for exercise is the increasing number of research studies verifying that exercise is helpful in the treatment of depression. Children are being diagnosed and treated for depression much more frequently than ever before. It also has been shown that obese children experience depression more than normal-weight children. In one study of over 50 children in a hospital-based weight-management program, the obese patients showed significant depression and lowered self-esteem (Sheslow).

A Duke University study of 156 individuals found that an exercise program of thirty minutes of brisk exercise three times a week is just as effective in relieving the symptoms of major depression as drug therapy. A six-month follow-up study showed that an ongoing exercise program greatly reduces the chances of the depression returning (Blumenthal). Numerous other studies verify the positive effects of exercise in the treatment of depression. Exercise has been shown to increase levels of serotonin, release endorphins (the body's mood-elevating and pain-relieving compounds), and reduce levels of cortisol, which is released by the adrenal gland during stress. Symptoms of depression in children can differ from symptoms in adults and require diagnosis and treatment by a health professional. Your pediatrician should definitely be consulted if you think that your child is depressed.

The American Heart Association recommends that all children age five and older should participate in at least thirty minutes of moderately intense activities (household chores, yard work, playground and neighborhood games) every day. It is also recommended that children should participate in at least thirty minutes of vigorous physical activities (jogging, biking, and competitive sports) at least three to four days each week. In spite of this need, studies indicate that fewer than one in four children get twenty minutes of vigorous activity every day of the week. A survey of over 17,000 adolescents revealed that only 21.3% of individuals in this age group participated in one or more days of physical education per week in their schools (Gordon-Larsen). Many obese children have difficulty beginning an exercise program. Therefore, we recommend that these children start with low-impact, less strenuous exercise, such as walking or biking.

Although congress passed a resolution twelve years ago to encourage state and local physical education daily for all schoolchildren, little progress has been made. The Physical Education for Progress (PEP) Act was introduced in the U.S. Senate in May 1999. If enacted, it will provide $400 million over a five-year period to improve physical education programs for all kindergarten through twelfth-grade students. The bill is co-sponsored by one-third of the members of the U.S. Senate. Parents should advocate for increased physical education programs in schools and encourage their children to engage in after-school sports or outdoor neighborhood activities with their friends. Inquiring about and supporting the school programs can help to accomplish this.

Children who participate in intense physical activity will benefit from the Sugar Busters way of eating. Before engaging in long-distance running or other strenuous physical activity, eating low-glycemic, complex carbohydrates is recommended and is necessary for the buildup of glycogen stores in the body. Glycogen is depleted during exercise or fasting. Consuming a low-glycemic meal before exercise causes more fat to be burned yet does not reduce the endurance capacity (Wee). Many people believe that sports drinks are essential during physical activity. The electrolytes and water in sports drinks are important to avoid dehydration and muscle cramps; however, sports drinks also usually contain large amounts of unnecessary sugar. Choose water or low-sugar sports drinks.

Activities that involve family members as a group in physical exercise can reinforce your focus on this important component of obesity and illness prevention. This means that you must find creative ways to promote family activities, whether it is a bike caravan, a hike through the city park, or family lawn and garden maintenance. Did you know that routine gardening offers excellent exercise for all parts of the body? Your family activity can be as ambitious as training together for a marathon or as low-key as a brisk walk around the neighborhood. Just remember to turn off that TV and computer and get moving!

10

The Terrible Trio

No children's book would be complete without a discussion of the "terrible twos." Well, we choose instead to discuss the "terrible threes." It would be great if we could point to three foods and say, "eliminate these foods from your child's diet and you will be triumphant in the battle against poor nutrition." Unfortunately, it is not that easy. You have learned about the tremendous importance of evaluating foods by using the glycemic index. This is a guide to live by or actually, to live longer by. It is your good-food bible. While all high-glycemic foods contribute to the problem of poor food choices, there are three high-glycemic foods that are consumed more frequently and in greater quantity by our children and should be avoided. The following foods are the Terrible Trio: **sugar-sweetened soft drinks, french fries, and candy.**

Think about it. How often do you see these foods marketed to kids, and how often do you see them in the hands and mouths of our children? They get our vote for the prime candidates in the Nasty Food Villain contest. Let's investigate the problems with each of the Terrible Trio.

The Center for Science in the Public Interest quotes some alarming facts about soft-drink consumption. In 1998, soft drinks accounted for more than one-third of all refined sugars in an American's diet. That was a ninefold increase since 1942, when the American Medical Association's Council on Foods and Nutrition recommended a restriction of the consumption of sugar in carbonated beverages and candy because of its low nutritional value. Currently, soft drinks are the largest single source of refined sugars in the diet of Americans (Jacobson).

What can soft drinks possibly add to the diet of our children but too much sugar and added calories that are poor substitutes for the needed calcium present in skim or low-fat milk? Americans now use soft drinks as a frequent snack and mealtime drink rather than an occasional treat. This unhealthy habit, combined with the billions of dollars companies spend in targeting young consumers, poses quite a challenge for parents to overcome in their efforts to encourage correct food choices.

Notice that no food labels contain information listing the amount of added sugar. The Center for Science in the Public Interest (CSPI) is a nonprofit research and advocacy group for consumers. CSPI is working diligently to promote the requirement that the amount of added sugar be required on packaging. Fortunately, the sugar content is provided on most soft drinks, which the CSPI refers to as liquid candy, and what a content it is!

Scientific data demonstrates that children ages six to eleven consume 91 grams of added caloric sweeteners per day. Added caloric sweeteners are all sugars that are not a natural part of the food. They are sugars that are added during home cooking or commercial food processing. The most common food sources with added sweeteners are soft drinks, candy, sweetened grains and cereals, and sweetened fruit drinks (Guthrie). Our recommendation is no more than 24 grams, or 6 teaspoons, of added sugar per day. What a difference between the 24 grams that we recommend and the 91 grams of added sugar that most children consume! Since most soft drinks contain between 38 and 45 grams of sugar, one soft drink contains double the amount of added sugar that should be consumed in one day. Because other sugars will inevitably be ingested each day, it is clear why we stress the avoidance of soft drinks.

Our second candidate for the Terrible Trio is worse than soda pop in some aspects. Teenagers consume more french-fried potatoes than any other vegetable. Take the high-glycemic index of white potatoes (95 on the average), add saturated fat for frying, and you have a formula for disaster. Potatoes have the highest glycemic index of any vegetable. The small amount of fiber they contain will not inhibit the spiked insulin curve that occurs after digestion. One serving of french fries can contain over 25 grams of fat and 50 grams of carbohydrates. A high-glycemic food cooked in high fat is *doubly* unhealthy. The combination of a high-glycemic food and a high-fat food should always be avoided. Consider the typical fast-food meal: a greasy hamburger on a white bun, french fries, and a soft drink. Things probably could not get any worse unless you finish the meal with candy for dessert.

Candy and other confections are all too frequently used to reward kids or to keep them quiet while we wheel them around the grocery store. So candy, a major source of empty calories for children, is our third candidate for the Terrible Trio. Foods that contain empty calories have no nutritional value and usually displace healthy foods from our diet. There was concern in the 1970s about sugar increasing hyperactive symptoms in susceptible children. Although there was never conclusive evidence to prove it, some parents report that candy or sugar causes their children to become hyper or agitated. More studies are needed to evaluate a possible connection between dietary sugars and hyperactivity. One positive thing is that we are seeing more teachers and parents advocating for wholesome snacks at school. This trend must continue. Regrettably, a recent survey of snacks served in twenty-four San Diego public middle schools showed that one-third of the snacks were candy. Over 88% of the snacks sold were high in fat and/or high in sugar (Wildey).

In order to increase their revenues, more and more schools are signing exclusive vending machine contracts with specific soft drink companies. Health advocates are becoming progressively more concerned about the effect these vending machines will have on America's schoolchildren (Kaufman). In addition to replacing milk in children's diets, the high sugar content and the lack of nutritional value in soft drinks offer only negative health consequences. This is a poor exchange for additional school revenue.

The Terrible Trio needs your attention. Just think of what positive results could come from a sweeping reduction of soft drinks, french fries, and candy in our children's diets. Often, we read in the newspaper or see on TV that a particular product designed and marketed for children is being recalled. The product might be an infant car seat, carrier, or even a crib. The products, for one reason or another, can be injurious to children. Have you ever heard of a recall of junk food, other than because it contained a contaminant? We would like to have a recall of foods that are high-glycemic carbohydrates or have high refined sugar content. Then we might be well on the way to curbing the obesity epidemic.

11

Parents as Advocates

Parents must take charge and become ardent advocates in all aspects of a revolutionary changeover to the Sugar Busters lifestyle. Since the change has to occur in many areas of your child's life, you have the challenge of taking on big business, the school system, the media, extended family, your child's peers, and your own home. Quite a task, you say; not really, and you can do it. Very little is being done to acknowledge worldwide obesity and resultant health crisis. Many parents are not recognizing the consequences of the crisis or their role in remediating it. Those who do often feel powerless to do anything about it. Your task is to acknowledge the serious consequences of poor food choices and lack of physical activity, then advocate for change in your own home and all other areas that impact your children's well-being. Your own influence should not be underestimated.

This is a war that can be won starting with little battles. Begin with advocacy in your own home. Parents should learn to take charge again. Bombarded for years by an ever-increasing usurping of home rule by the media, advertising, and peer pressure, parental influence began slipping away. The movement for parents to regain authority and influence appears to be gaining momentum. The effectiveness of parents' frank communication with their children on such topics as drugs, sexuality, and violence seems to be making a difference.

Until recently we may not have had an argument for the importance of parents' role in influencing the nutrition of their children. There are too many other urgent things to worry about: school performance, drugs, family communication, and social interaction. While parents were attending to all of these other pressing issues, researchers were quietly and diligently working on another growing concern: the adverse effects of poor diet on the health of children. Suddenly, we are confronted with the startling truth that the matter of nutrition can no longer be left to simmer on the back burner. Unless we get fired up on the topic, the problem will only continue to grow.

It cannot be expected that a Sugar Busters lifestyle can become a household routine immediately. Going "cold turkey" might be the ideal, but everyone knows habits are hard to break. We ask parents to strive for the ideal, but above all we want success. Good nutrition isn't built in one day. To achieve success we recommend a phase-in period of gradually substituting Sugar Busters food for the sugar-laden, high-glycemic carbohydrates that your children have become accustomed to eating.

Don't Give Up!

An important thing to remember is: Don't give up! One study, reported in the *American Academy of Pediatrics' Guide to Your Child's Nutrition*, indicated that children did not accept a new food until it had been presented to them on an average of ten times (Dietz). Let us say that the new food introduced has to appear and then reappear as if by magic and without a hassle. It's best to avoid a standoff because a power struggle can sabotage your best efforts to effect change.

Reframing

Since you are a role model for your child, let us consider your own attitude about the Sugar Busters way of eating. The way you feel about following any eating regimen, a good one (Sugar Busters) or a not-so-good one (diets or junk food), will influence your own child's attitude. Remember that Sugar Busters is considered a way of eating rather than a diet. You frequently hear that people on diets feel that they are deprived, that they have difficulty being consistent, and that they cannot wait until they lose enough weight to be able to go off the awful diet.

It is time for all of us to **reframe** our thinking about what we eat. Reframing is a process that therapists use to help to change the way one views a particular situation. Let's use a common example. Consider a glass that has liquid up to its midpoint. A pessimist (unhopeful person) will bemoan the fact that the glass is **half empty**. An optimist (hopeful person) will come along and encourage the pessimist to look at the glass as **half full. Now, consider how you might reframe your way of eating.** You can think, "I feel depressed and deprived because, with my weight problem, I will have to diet for the rest of my life. If I don't diet to maintain my normal weight, I will be at risk for heart disease, high blood pressure, and diabetes. I have so many other problems in my life that the thought of dieting discourages and depresses me. Why do I have to give up the things that I enjoy like cake, candy, soft drinks, and french fries?"

Or you can think, "My, how the diet of humans has changed over the past decades corresponding with the high rate of obesity. Is it healthy for me to consume 150 pounds of added refined sugar a year as well as highly refined processed foods? Do I want to continue to substitute junk foods for the cancer- and cholesterol-fighting substances found in fruits, vegetables, and whole grains? Do I really need fast food, or is it a convenience and a habit? Is eating the correct foods that maintain low insulin levels and provide essential disease-fighting nutrients just a diet, or is it really saving my life?" If you can change your attitude about eating from the first scenario to the second, you will provide your child with a role model who uses food as a way of nurturing the body rather than placing it at risk for serious disease.

Your first challenge is to take charge of the nutrition in your own household with a great deal of enthusiasm. Slowly introduce Sugar Busters foods such as whole-grain breads, brown rice, unsweetened drinks, and unsweetened cereals. Remember that the Sugar Busters lifestyle is about making healthy choices of foods that will not raise insulin and blood-sugar levels. The meal plans, recipes, and product suggestions in this book will help you accomplish this. It is extremely important to use a phase-in stage so that new foods can be introduced gradually and eventually be substituted for the high-sugar, over-processed junk foods that so many children are consuming so frequently and in such large amounts.

All children go through stages during which they will eat only one kind of food. Remember that it is important to introduce and reintroduce the correct foods, even disguising the food in a variety of different recipes. Hide those black beans, for example, in a whole-wheat pita pocket with lettuce, salsa, and cheese. Power struggles over food should be avoided because given enough variety, children can learn to eat a diet rich in proper choices. Do you realize the control that you have over these correct food choices? How many children do the family grocery shopping? Not many! Since you have the buying power, it follows that you can be the decision maker. Fill your kitchen storage baskets with fresh fruits, rinse out the cookie jar and use it to store nuts or unsweetened cereals. Substitution is the key because no one goes hungry following the Sugar Busters lifestyle.

Issues that lead to eating disorders can begin early in childhood. These problems occur predominantly in girls. Media attention on extreme thinness as an ideal magnifies the dilemma. This fixation is both unhealthy and unrealistic. If a parent adds to this pressure, the problem is compounded. Accordingly, you should be very cautious in the kind of approach you use in dealing with your child's weight problem.

Children who are overweight frequently have to deal with low self-esteem and the negative and hurtful comments of their peers. Who is more aware of this than you, the parent? And who is more responsive to this than a parent who has been a target of similar hurt as an overweight child, adolescent, and then adult? Your role as an advocate is essential. Take an assertive rather than an aggressive approach. One way of doing this is to use **"I"** rather than accusing **"you"** statements. Instead of **"you** always eat the wrong foods" say, "**I** am going to buy a lot of good food choices for this family." Advocacy for your child can center on developing a family team effort to foster a spirit of mutual encouragement and support such as, "In this home we eat a lot of healthy foods."

Taking charge of the nutritional needs of your household also means taking charge of the TV, computer, and video games. It is estimated that American children are spending approximately five hours a day in these sedentary kinds of activities. We recommend that you limit your child's "couch potato" time to two hours a day. An American Heart Association study indicated that children who reduced their TV viewing also reduced their BMI (Body Mass Index). Combine inactivity with snacking or dining in front of the TV and you have a recipe for weight gain. So we also recommend that children not be allowed to eat in front of the TV.

Dining Together as a Family

When a daughter of one of the authors was in middle school about eight years ago, the principal commented that she believed the decrease in frequency of families dining together had a direct relationship to the lowered vocabulary scores that were occurring on school standardized tests. "Families," she said, "don't spend much time conversing with each other anymore." What an interesting observation.

While we are not aware of any research on the issue of family dining and vocabulary scores, we know the results of an important study funded by grants from the National Institutes of Health and Harvard Medical School. The study involved over 17,000 boys and girls aged nine to fourteen years and investigated the relationship between the frequency of eating together as a family and the quality of the children's diets. The researchers concluded that "eating family dinner together was associated with healthful dietary intake patterns, including more fruits and vegetables, less fried food and soda, less saturated and trans-fats, lower glycemic load, more fiber and micronutrients from food, and no material differences in red meat or snack food"

(Gillman). As can be expected, older children ate dinner with the family less frequently. Eighty-eight percent of the mothers in the survey were employed, yet that fact did not change the frequency of eating dinner together as a family. It was reported that during family dinners, nutritional topics were often discussed.

What better time to guide children to the correct food choices and reinforce and encourage good lifetime eating habits than at the dinner table? In our hurried times, a commitment to this daily face-to-face interaction with our children can have much more than nutritional benefits. Who knows, those vocabulary scores may also climb.

Now that you have gained control of nutrition in your home, you can tackle the rest of the world. Of course you cannot do it alone, but if enough people who read this book choose to voice their opinions and make their demands known, eventually there will be a change. You should become an advocate for the proper food choices and adequate physical education programs at your child's school. This includes awareness of school lunch menus and the types of snacks that are offered. We know of an instance where parents were instrumental in removing a candy cart that was being wheeled around the school loaded with pounds of sugary snacks for sale. If your child's school does not provide a selection of low-glycemic carbohydrates for lunch, then your child should be able to bring lunch from home.

Too often we hear complaints that grocery stores and restaurants are not providing foods essential for the Sugar Busters lifestyle. It is time you learned about consumer power. Here is an example of that power. One of the authors was asked to give a Sugar Busters presentation to a medical convention in Alabama. The audience discussion turned to the problems of a hectic lifestyle and the inevitable trip to a fast-food restaurant because of too many activities and too little time. Audience members voiced concern that there are very few menu choices in takeout food restaurants. One parent spoke out, saying that the only local restaurant in her small town is an internationally known, fast-food drive through. She said that she had repeatedly asked for the addition of some Sugar Buster–friendly foods. To her surprise, on a recent visit to the drive through, whole-wheat buns had been added to the menu! It is doubtful that the buns were 100% whole wheat but even a gradual change indicates progress.

Another example of the consumer's influence on change is occurring in New Orleans, home of the Sugar Busters authors, and the initial grassroots Sugar Busters movement. Since the publication of *Sugar Busters! Cut Sugar to Trim Fat,* restaurants throughout the city and neighboring cities and states have altered their menus to include Sugar Busters foods. You will see bread trays filled with whole-wheat rolls, and sweet potatoes substituted for white potatoes. Even the Asian restaurants are offering brown rice.

Don't hesitate to make your food choices known to restaurants and grocers. Have you noticed that some cereal and bread manufacturers are now including a no-sugar-added phrase on their packaging? Similarly, we are seeing more stone-ground wheat and fiber claims on labels. So, when you ask us, "Where can we get Sugar Busters foods?" we have a simple answer. The principle is supply and demand. You demand and they will supply.

Behavior Modification

You can support your child's efforts to adjust to the Sugar Busters way of eating by using behavior-modification techniques. Make copies of the chart at the end of this chapter and post one each week in a prominent place in your home. Use the charts to record your child's daily and weekly progress.

Behavior modification is a method used to alter behavior patterns. In the plan we are suggesting, you use positive reinforcement (rewards) when your child makes correct nutrition and behavior choices. Young children (ages five to eight) need to be reinforced more frequently than older children (ages nine to twelve). You may want to reward younger children daily and older children weekly. You know your child and therefore should choose the frequency of reward that you think will be most effective.

You are also the best judge of the kind of reward that will be most appropriate. However, **do not give food as a reward.** We recommend other inexpensive rewards. Young children may like stickers, art materials, trips to the movies, or special activities with parents. Intangible rewards such as child-parent activities can be very effective.

Using the behavior chart as a visual reminder is a great reinforcer for behavioral change. The chart also gives a child the opportunity to follow his or her progress. Positive results may require some time. In fact, your child may show some initial regression with this method. It is important to persist in encouraging your child to continue. When your child begins to experience positive results, the success will become its own reward. Positive behavior will be learned and tangible rewards can possibly be phased out. Here again, you can be the judge of what is most effective for your own child.

Figure 4: Sugar Busters Behavior-Modification Chart

Child's Name:

Activity	Points	Mon	Tue	Wed	Thu	Fri	Sat	Sun
Whole-grain cereal	10							
Whole-grain bread (only 2 slices)	10							
Fruit or veggie snack	10							
No soft drinks	20							
Exercise 30 minutes	10							
No eating while watching TV	10							
Limit TV to 2 hours/day	10							
No fast food	20							
No sugary snacks or desserts	20							
6 glasses water a day	2 points per glass							
No bedtime snack	10							
TOTAL DAILY POINTS								

Parents may give non-food rewards for points. List rewards.

60 points per day _____

80 points per day _____

120 points per day _____

12

How to Determine if a Child Is Overweight

You cannot always tell simply by their appearance if children are overweight or obese. Since the weights of adults and children have increased dramatically over the past few decades, parents may think that they and their children are of normal weight when in fact they are overweight. As populations become heavier together, the perception of what is normal weight changes. The Body Mass Index (BMI) is a standardized tool to determine the amount of body fat both in adults and children.

The Body Mass Index is a calculation of a person's weight relative to his height. The BMI is calculated by dividing the weight in kilograms by the height in meters squared: the formula is Kg/M^2 where Kg is the weight in kilograms and M is the height in meters. It has been used extensively to determine if adults or children are overweight or obese. We will demonstrate several ways to determine your child's BMI. A BMI equal to or greater than 25 in adults indicates that the adult is overweight. A BMI equal to or greater than 30 indicates obesity. As the BMI increases to above 25, the risk of complications from overweight also increases.

In addition to determining whether a child is overweight or obese, the BMI is very useful in determining if a child is underweight or normal weight. Since the weights and heights of children change with age, the BMI changes until growth is completed. In children the BMI changes as the child grows taller and gains weight. In adults, since height is fixed, the BMI changes only with weight.

The Centers for Disease Control has gathered data on children relative to height and weight (BMI). We rely on percentiles of data from the Centers for Disease Control to determine overweight and obesity. These percentiles rank children according to BMI and age: the greater the weight, the higher the percentile.

A child with a BMI equal to or greater than the 85th percentile is considered to be overweight. Any child with a BMI equal to, or greater than, the 95th percentile is considered to be obese, and this obesity is very likely to persist into adulthood. The percentage of children in the U.S. who are overweight is approximately 25%. This means that 25% of children will have a BMI that exceeds the 85th percentile when matched for age and sex.

Although the BMI charts and percentiles are very useful for measuring body fat, some overweight children may be misclassified as normal weight. Conversely, a small percentage of upper-limit normal weight children could be misclassified as overweight. For instance, some athletic, muscular children may have a normal amount of body fat, yet have a high BMI. It also has been noted that children who are very inactive may have a normal BMI, but an unhealthy amount of body fat. In spite of these limitations, the BMI is considered to be extremely useful in identifying weight problems in most children.

We suggest three ways to determine your child's BMI.

First, you can ask your pediatrician to determine your child's BMI. The pediatrician has access to tables to determine the BMI for all ages. Then you can refer to our tables to determine the percentile ranking.

Second, you can calculate the BMI. The formula is Weight/Height/Height × 703. Divide the weight in pounds by the height in inches and divide by the height in inches again. Multiply the results by 703. For example, if the weight is 140 pounds and the height is 60 inches, the calculation would be as follows: 140/60 = 2.33, 2.33/60 = .0388, .0388 × 703 = 27.2764. The BMI = 27.

You can use the calculator at the Centers for Disease Control's

Web site to calculate the BMI. This is found on the Internet at *www.cdc.gov/nccdphp/dnpa/bmi/calc-bmi.htm*.

You can use either the English calculator or the metric calculator.

After you determine the child's BMI, locate the appropriate chart for your child's gender at the end of this chapter. Find your child's BMI number in the column on the left. Locate your child's age on the bottom of the chart and move up until you reach and intersect your child's BMI. That intersecting point will indicate the percentile found on the right side of the chart. If the percentile is 85 or greater, your child is overweight. If the percentile is 95 or greater, your child is considered to be obese and should be evaluated by your pediatrician for a planned weight-loss program. Some children falling between the 85th percentile and the 95th percentile who maintain that weight, may grow into their weight as they grow taller. This means that as the child grows taller and if the weight remains the same, the child will lose body fat. The BMI will then decrease as the child grows. However, even though this normalization of weight may eventually occur, you should not ignore early warning signs that your child may be at risk for developing obesity. The Sugar Busters way of eating will help children achieve and maintain a normal weight.

Figure 5.
CDC Growth Charts: United States

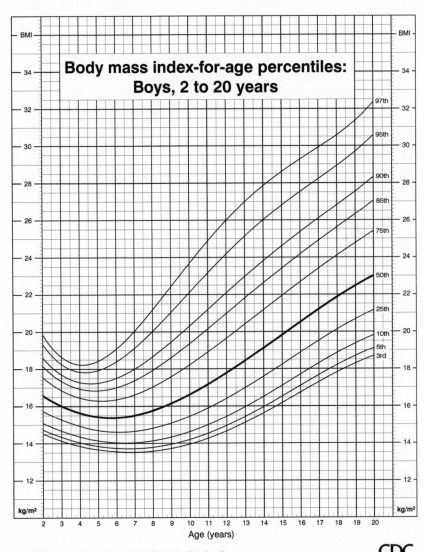

Body mass index-for-age percentiles:
Boys, 2 to 20 years

SOURCE: Developed by the National Center for Health Statistics in collaboration with
the National Center for Chronic Disease Prevention and Health Promotion (2000).

CDC

Figure 6.
CDC Growth Charts: United States

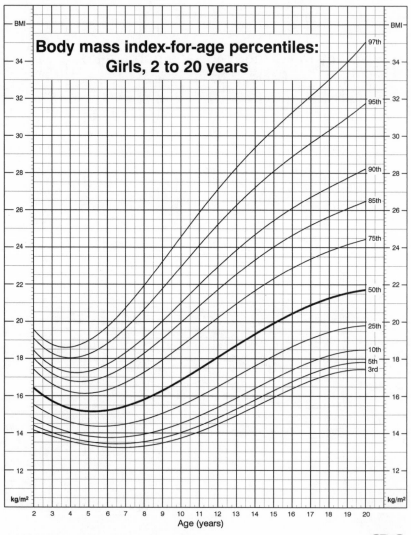

**Body mass index-for-age percentiles:
Girls, 2 to 20 years**

SOURCE: Developed by the National Center for Health Statistics in collaboration with
the National Center for Chronic Disease Prevention and Health Promotion (2000).

13

Research Survey and Analysis

During the writing of *Sugar Busters for Kids*, we developed and posted a questionnaire on our Web site. We were attempting to determine whether there is a difference in the foods consumed by normal weight and overweight children, with a focus on specific foods and fast-food consumption. The survey was also designed to investigate the kinds of foods children are eating, whether or not they are on Sugar Busters, their ease of adjusting to Sugar Busters, and what, if any, success is being achieved. The survey does not reflect the general population because it does not represent a cross section of the United States population. Answers came from parents who chose to reply to our Web site questionnaire.

The response was great and the results were very significant. Over 106 questionnaires were answered and e-mailed to us by parents. We learned that children respond to the Sugar Busters way of eating and have just as much success as do their parents.

Before we give you an analysis of the results, here are some very informative comments from the parents who responded. One mom who had been on Sugar Busters for one year reported that she had lost twenty-seven pounds. Her husband and daughter lost fifteen pounds each. The family eliminated sugary foods like candy and cake. They also eliminated potatoes, carrots, and some very high-sugar fruits. They substituted rye bread for white bread and cut down on pastas and rice. They eliminated all sugar colas and substituted two diet drinks per day. Snacks now consist of string cheese, rye crackers, cheese, and peanuts. The family does not eat fast foods. When they dine out, they order turkey sandwiches on whole-wheat bread and ask for fruit instead of fries. Mom had this to say about her daughter's success: "She is incredible on Sugar Busters! She has really gotten used to it and can eat more and remain a great weight. This is truly a miracle for all of us who have had to watch our weight all of our life. I wish I had known about this years ago. My struggle with my weight would not have existed."

Another family responded that they eliminated a lot of refined sugar snacks, white breads, white pastas, and potatoes. The child, age eleven, now enjoys whole-wheat bread, eats more fruit and "icees," which are made from fruit. Now portion sizes can be cut down because she gets full much quicker. After four months on the Sugar Busters way of eating, Mom has lost thirty pounds, Dad has lost twenty-two, and the child has lost fifteen. Mom commented, "Sugar Busters has completely changed my family's way of thinking and of enjoying foods. It has brought us closer, eating as a family and sharing our weight-loss accomplishments as a family." This testimonial confirms what we believe. A child's success on Sugar Busters is related to the parents' role as a model and a participant. Success can really be a family affair.

With few exceptions, either one or both parents in families answering the survey described themselves as overweight. We detected from parents' comments that they are very concerned about future weight problems in their child even if the child is not currently overweight. Their concern is justified because we know that children of overweight parents are at high risk to become overweight themselves.

Perception and Diagnosis

Our survey concluded that many parents do not recognize that their children are overweight or obese when they actually are. From data reported by parents on each child's height, weight, age, and sex, we calculated the child's BMI and percentile. Parents were asked if they considered their child to be overweight and if the child had been diagnosed as being overweight. Using the percentile we calculated for each child, we determined that 50% of the children who are overweight are not recognized as such by the parent. More surprising is that 15% of parents of obese children (95th percentile or above) do not even consider their children to be overweight. In our survey, 77% of overweight children were not diagnosed as overweight. Forty percent of obese children in the survey were not diagnosed as being overweight.

These findings raise two serious concerns. One is that parents are not recognizing that their children are overweight or obese. The second concern is that the weight problem is not being diagnosed, and therefore not being treated. Failure to identify the problem will only perpetuate the obesity epidemic.

The survey listed different foods, and questions were asked to determine the frequency of consumption of the foods. Let's first look at the popularity of the Terrible Trio:

Soft Drinks

Of the overweight or obese children in our survey, 53% consumed soft drinks every day. Only 29% of normal-weight children consumed soft drinks daily; 43% of normal-weight children reportedly never consume soft drinks.

French Fries

Of overweight children in the survey, 81% regularly consume french fries, while 51% of normal-weight children consume french fries.

Candy

Of overweight and obese children in the study, 90% consume candy either daily or several times a week. Of normal-weight children, 71% consume candy either daily or several times a week.

Our survey illustrates that there is a significant difference in the percentage of overweight children who consume soft drinks, french fries, and candy. We also learned that both normal and overweight children are consuming fast food; however, there is a difference in the two groups. Of overweight children, 100% consume fast food several times a week, while 82% of normal-weight children consume fast-food several times a week.

Results of the questionnaire are clear. A higher percentage of overweight children are consuming soft drinks, french fries, candy, and fast food.

Our research also indicated other poor food choices of overweight children. These included white bread, white rice, potatoes, chips, cookies, sugar-sweetened cereals, and whole milk.

Comparison of Food Consumption

Food	Normal Weight Child	Overweight or Obese Child
Candy	71%	90%
French fries	51%	81%
Soft drinks	29%	53%
Fast food	82%	100%

Healthy Food Choices

Analysis of the data also showed a large variation among the children in consumption of two very healthy foods: fish and beans. Fish are high in omega-3 fatty acids and act to lower cholesterol. The American Heart Association is now recommending that everyone eat two 3-ounce servings of fatty fish, such as salmon, sardines, or herring each week. Beans are an important source of dietary fiber. Of the normal-weight children in our survey, 42% eat fish and beans; 73% of normal-weight children eat fish and/or beans. Only 54% of overweight and obese children in our survey eat fish or beans; 46% of overweight children do not consume either fish or beans.

Comparison of Healthy Food Consumption

Food	Normal Weight Child	Overweight or Obese Child
Fish	56%	43%
Beans	53%	43%
Fish and Beans	42%	20%
Neither	27%	46%

Parents' Comments

The parent-comment section of the survey enabled us to identify parents' concerns about their children's weight, eating habits, and self-esteem. Parents who are overweight are concerned that their children, whether they are overweight or not, will have to deal with the same problems that they had throughout their lives.

Some parents are worried that their children's terrible snacking habits will lead to obesity and health disorders. Parents who are diabetic are concerned that their children will develop diabetes and they feel that it makes sense to modify their children's way of eating now. They are right to be concerned, because risk factors, which include obesity and consumption of high-glycemic carbohydrates, can lead to the development of Type 2 diabetes.

The survey revealed that parents are successful in adopting the Sugar Busters way of eating to family life when they use a phase-in period of substituting correct foods for unhealthy foods. Many parents who follow the Sugar Busters method hope that their children will eventually make correct food choices when they eat away from home. They now prepare their children's school lunches themselves and offer suggestions to their children about better food choices at fast-food restaurants.

Parents also listed foods that were easier for their children to adjust to, as well as those that were more difficult. Whole-wheat bread, brown rice, fruit, sweet potatoes, and ice cream without added sugar were easiest to integrate into the diet. Children found that whole-wheat pasta and vegetables were the most difficult of the recommended foods to accept.

Everyone reporting found success with Sugar Busters. Overweight children lost weight on Sugar Busters. Obese children lost up to fifteen pounds after a few months on Sugar Busters. Without exception, the children who were not overweight maintained their normal weight. Many parents started Sugar Busters before their children. The survey revealed all children on Sugar Busters had one or both parents on Sugar Busters. We know that children do better on weight-loss programs when the whole family is following the program.

Results of our research survey clearly indicated that the parents who responded are concerned about the kinds of foods that their children are consuming as well as the risks of childhood obesity. Many parents have found success with the Sugar Busters way of eating and choose it as a plan for the entire family. Other parents ask for help and are searching for a plan that is practical, logical, and reasonable. Those who have tried it agree that Sugar Busters is that plan.

14

Summary:
Sugar Busters and Kids

You have learned the importance of substituting low-glycemic carbohydrates for high-glycemic carbohydrates. You also have learned the significance of a diet rich in whole grains and fiber for its protective characteristics and for weight control. The value of regular exercise has been stressed. In addition, we discussed the importance of your role as an advocate in ensuring that your child is gradually given the correct food choices at home and school. Now we will focus on other recommendations to help you incorporate Sugar Busters into your family's lifestyle. Now that you are equipped with the knowledge of how and why Sugar Busters works, the following details of how to implement this way of eating will help you to easily make Sugar Busters a part of your everyday life.

Your Pediatrician as a Resource

Your pediatrician or family doctor is the best resource for monitoring your child's weight, growth, and development. Your child's doctor should supervise any weight-loss program to ensure adequate intake of calcium, nutrients, and vitamins. After taking a medical history, giving a physical examination, and evaluating the results of any appropriate tests, your pediatrician can determine whether or not your child may be in the 10% of the overweight children who have endocrine problems or genetic causes of obesity. A multivitamin and calcium supplement should be taken when a child is on any weight-loss program. Studies show that markedly obese children who achieve long-term weight loss may have a decrease in bone-mineral density (Willi). Young women who have decreased bone-mineral density may have osteoporosis later in life. Your pediatrician can give specific supplement recommendations.

General Guidelines

We do not recommend counting calories, because restricting calories during the weight management of overweight children rarely succeeds (Diamond). High-glycemic carbohydrates, such as white bread and potatoes, are one of the major causes of obesity.

Food should not be used as a reward. For example, do not allow fast food or junk food as an incentive for progress or as a prize for making good food choices. Neither should your child be punished for failing to stay with a weight-loss program. Use a phase-in period to gradually introduce the foods that we recommend. Substitute the correct food choices for the unhealthy ones over a period of weeks.

How to Be a Successful Sugar Busters Kid

Consume low- to moderate-glycemic carbohydrates instead of high-glycemic carbohydrates. Use the glycemic index as your constant guide to choose the foods you eat most frequently. This does not mean that you never can eat a ripe banana (GI 70), or a slice of watermelon (GI 77). (In general as fruits ripen the glycemic index increases.) Eat them as occasional foods or use them as a garnish. We recommend that you choose carbohydrates that have a glycemic index below 70. The lower the better when you are attempting to lose weight. Conversely, you should not consume excessive quantities of low-glycemic carbohydrates at one meal because you will then convert a low-glycemic meal into a high-glycemic meal because of glycemic load. Glycemic load is the product of grams of carbohydrate multiplied by the glycemic index. For example, brown rice has a glycemic index of 55. If you consume ½ cup, or 50 grams, of cooked brown rice, the glycemic index will be 55. If you consume 1 cup, or 100 grams, then the glycemic index in effect becomes 110. Therefore, overconsumption of *any* food is unhealthy.

Avoid the consumption of a high-glycemic food together with a high-fat food. Both carbohydrates and fats are sources of energy, the fuel for our bodies. The consumption of high-glycemic carbohydrates stimulates a greater insulin release, encourages the storage of sugar as fat, and prevents fat breakdown. The addition of a high-fat food to the high-glycemic food compounds the problem of fat storage because the dietary fat is also stored. An example of this is eating a steak (high-fat food) with a potato (high-glycemic carbohydrate). Consumption of a hamburger and french fries together or corn flakes and whole milk together are also combinations to avoid.

Limit your intake of added sugar to 24 grams or 6 teaspoons a day. This does not include the natural sugars found in fruit and milk, but the sugars you add to coffee, tea, recipes, and those found in commercially prepared foods and drinks. The body does not need added sugar; all the sugar that is needed can be obtained from natural sugars. Remember that just one soft drink contains 39 grams of sugar—more than our total daily recommendation.

Eat three meals and two snacks each day. It is important to distribute food consumption throughout the day and not overeat at any meal. When overeating occurs, as it usually does at the evening meal, the body goes into a storage mode. Combined with inactivity (sleep) this causes the food to be stored as fat rather than burned as fuel. Most of the cholesterol in the body is manufactured at night during sleep, so also avoid snacking after supper.

Limit portion sizes. It is a fact that restaurants are enlarging the plate sizes. Soft-drink bottles have also been enlarged from 6 ounces to 20 ounces. What has become the norm in restaurants is becoming the norm in homes. Carefully observe portion sizes on the labels of canned and packaged foods. We suggest that you especially avoid "all you can eat" restaurants and buffets. Why put yourself in this tempting situation?

Avoid all fruit drinks with added sugar. Limit fruit juice to one drink containing 100% fruit juice per day.

Whole fruit is preferable to fruit juice. Whole fruit has more fiber and a lower glycemic index than fruit juice. For example, an orange has a glycemic index of 43, while orange juice has a glycemic index of 57. We think that consumers have become more aware of the difference between drinks that are labeled fruit drinks, yet contain large amounts of sugar and very little fruit, and drinks that contain 100% fruit. Refer to our section on reading labels in Part II for information that will help you to choose packaged foods wisely.

Consume three servings of whole grains a day. Consume 30 to 35 grams of fiber a day.

Whole-grain and fiber-rich foods lower the glycemic index and provide both nutrients and satiety. It is essential that these foods become an integral part of our way of eating, because too many children are consuming nutritionally poor carbohydrates. Cakes, cookies, candy, and soft drinks are high in sugar, yet offer little nutrition. These high-glycemic carbohydrates displace healthy foods such as whole grains and fiber in the diet.

Drink water, skim or 1% milk, or unsweetened tea. Avoid all sugar-sweetened soft drinks. Limit diet drinks to one or two per day.

We recommend a drink that is inexpensive, sugarless, healthy, essential, and crystal clear: **water**. You should drink six to eight glasses of water each day. We can assure you that if you begin substituting water for soft drinks at meals, over time the soft drinks will not be missed. The health benefits of green tea are well known and children can learn to enjoy unsweetened tea. Skim or 1% milk is recommended because of its lower overall fat content and especially because of its lower saturated-fat content. Here again, you will find that it is easy to adjust to low-fat milk.

Avoid fast food and the most frequently consumed problem foods: desserts, candy, white bread, white rice, potatoes, and sweetened soft drinks.

Of the overweight children in our survey, 100% consumed fast foods regularly. We recommend that you read Part II of this book to learn how to prepare your own nutritious "fast foods."

Exercise regularly.

Exercise is a very effective way to make insulin more efficient and therefore lower insulin levels. Exercise works in conjunction with the Sugar Busters way of eating to prevent and eliminate fat storage in the body.

Parents should act as advocates.

What has been done to the diets of our children? Quite simply, fiber has been removed; high fat has been replaced with high sugar. Our children sit for hours inactive in front of TVs eating from oversized plates filled with poor food choices, while they watch commercials that encourage consumption of more of the same. When is the last time you have seen a commercial for spinach or broccoli? So you have to be the producer of infomercials in your home that target appropriate food choices.

Your role as an advocate begins with learning the principles of a healthy way of eating, then phasing in correct food choices, substituting correct choices for poor eating habits, and maintaining an ongoing commitment to the Sugar Busters way of eating. Forget dieting! Sugar Busters is a way of life. This way of life is easier than you may think, but it will not happen for your family without your own dedication and your own spirit of enthusiasm. Present Sugar Busters as a family affair. Unlike many diets, in which parents are on a weight-loss plan eating one way, and the children are eating something else, the Sugar Busters way of eating can (and should) include the whole family. Why shouldn't all family members benefit from good nutrition?

Part II

Shopping, Cooking, and Eating Sugar Busters Style

15

How to Shop and Cook Sugar Busters Style

There is one remarkable characteristic about Sugar Buster followers: their enthusiasm. We see this enthusiasm when we give presentations on the Sugar Busters concept, at book signings, from comments on the Web site, from patients, and in letters from many individuals. Sugar Busters have this zeal because the Sugar Busters lifestyle is not a dreaded challenge, as are most "diets." The enthusiasm comes simply from the great results obtained, the ease in understanding the concept, and the effortlessness in adapting to this way of eating. Now that you have an understanding of the Sugar Busters concept, it is time to apply what you have learned to shopping, cooking, and eating the Sugar Busters way.

Filling your grocery cart and stocking your pantry with the correct choices requires careful thought because package labeling can be very deceptive. Learning to read labels will be your first challenge; however, it is one that is easily met. Then learning to cook Sugar Busters style can be as simple as you choose to make it. Why? Because you can easily learn to substitute colorful fresh fruits and vegetables, fiber, and whole grains for the highly processed, high-glycemic carbohydrates that you may be accustomed to eating. In addition to helping you maintain a normal weight, many of these foods have the added benefit of protecting against cancer and heart disease. We will give you a list of our favorite foods and tell you why we think they are so important.

You can learn to substitute spices for the heavy sauces that add weight both to your plates and your middle. And, believe it or not, you need not choose between fast food and hours of toiling over a hot stove. Simple food preparation can be healthy preparation. We want to propose some ideas that will help you while you are *in* the kitchen, so that you can get *out* of the kitchen *faster*.

A Lesson in Reading Labels

It is necessary to learn how to read food labels in order to make correct food choices. The information on the label will enable you to evaluate the macronutrient (carbohydrate, fat, and protein) content of the food. The label information will also guide you in determining the degree of processing of the carbohydrates, the amount of sugar, and the presence of less-known additives that can raise the glycemic index. After you have evaluated these characteristics of the food, you can then determine if the food fits into a Sugar Busters meal plan.

First, it is important to note the serving size listed on the label. Keep in mind, for example, that if the serving size is one-half cup and you consume one cup, you must double all of the amounts listed on the label to arrive at the total amount of sugar, fat, and so on that you are consuming.

Next, the grams per serving of the macronutrients are listed. Remember that the macronutrient content indicates the carbohydrate, fat, and protein composition of the food. Evaluate these ingredients to determine how well they fit into a daily meal plan that will meet the Sugar Busters recommended balanced diet for children of 50% carbohydrates, 30% fat, and 20% protein.

While examining the ingredient list, keep in mind that the ingredients are listed from the largest amount of an ingredient to the smallest. This is how you can determine if the claims listed on the box and in advertisements are legitimate. For example, the front of a box of crackers may claim they are "whole wheat!" prominently. However, when you read the label you may find "enriched wheat flour." Every Sugar Buster should know that "enriched wheat flour" is highly processed flour that is high on the glycemic index. Whole-grain wheat may be listed way down—even last on the list. The low listing indicates that the product actually contains very little whole grains, and in this case, the description "whole-wheat crackers" is deceptive. As you can see, this claim is definitely misleading the public.

Unless you learn to read labels and understand manufacturers' deliberate attempts to confuse consumers, you cannot become a knowledgeable Sugar Buster shopper. Be aware that unbleached wheat flour and enriched wheat flour are highly processed and could have as high a glycemic index as white flour. Look for products with stone-ground wheat listed as the first ingredient.

Another example of misleading food labels concerns the listing of the product's sugar content. There is no regulation requiring manufacturers to list the amount of added sugars as a separate item. Sugar is listed as the total sugar content. The consumer is not informed that sugar may have been included in *addition to* the natural sugar content of the product. There is no way to know what portion of sugar is natural and what is added. For instance, orange juice has natural sugar; however, many manufacturers have added sugars to the natural product during the processing. You now understand why it is so important to compare labels on different brands when shopping.

The Center for Science in the Public Interest is attempting to mandate the listing of added sugars on labels. The organization's director, Michael Jacobson, believes that "it's vital that food labels give consumers the information they need to reduce their consumption of added sugars."

We remind you again that when a manufacturer removes the fat from a product, sugar is frequently added. The blueberries in low-fat blueberry yogurt contribute very little to the sugar content. Do not be fooled. You will read on the ingredient list that sugar has a higher ranking than the blueberries. The public is led to believe that they are consuming the sugar in the natural fruit when, in fact, additional sugar has been added. Be selective because brands vary. Choose products with the least sugar.

Added sugar is not all you need to be concerned about. What about hidden sugar? The following ingredients can appear on the label and are forms of sugar, but do not appear as sugar on the label: malto-dextrin, dextrose, honey, malted barley, high-fructose corn syrup, syrup solids, hydrolyzed rice starch, corn starch, molasses, isomalt, and malt syrup. Remember that the inclusion of any of these items in the product just means more sugar for you to consume.

While reading labels is one way to learn how to make correct food choices, there is another, easier way. Buy lots of foods without labels. Load up your shopping cart with more foods found around the perimeter of the grocery store. These are fresh-food choices that obviously won't contain the added sugars found in canned, packaged, and processed foods. Most people do not consume the recommended daily allowance of fresh fruits and vegetables. These foods are readily available, quick to prepare, and do not require label reading.

Breakfast, Lunch, and Dinner Choices

Breakfast is an extremely important meal that must not be skipped! Several studies of children link poor school performance with not eating breakfast (Meyers). Missing breakfast can also lead to nutritional shortages that are not made up at other meals (Ohlson). The doctors who authored this book agree that most of the overweight and obese patients they treat report that they frequently skip breakfast. These observations certainly highlight the importance of breakfast. And of course, it is not enough to just *eat* breakfast; you must also consider *what* you eat for breakfast. This meal is the perfect time for whole-grain foods.

You learned earlier that children who consume a low-glycemic, high-fiber breakfast are less hungry between breakfast and lunch and also consume less food at lunch (Ludwig). If you want your children to start the day ready to learn, filled with the proper nutrients to keep them satisfied until lunch, then give them a low-glycemic, whole-grain breakfast. Remember that most children are consuming much less than the recommended daily intake of whole grains.

We are finally seeing an increase in the number of low-sugar, whole-grain cereals on the market. Is it because of popular demand? Certainly there are many more low-sugar, whole-grain cereals available than before *Sugar Busters! Cut Sugar to Trim Fat* became so popular. We recommend that you choose cereals that have no more than 5 grams of sugar per serving size, and the less sugar the better. Consider your role as a consumer and advocate. If you continue to ask for and buy unsweetened or less-sweetened cereals, more will appear on the grocery shelves. Hopefully one day these cereals will replace the hundreds of heavily sweetened varieties that are adding too many sugar grams to our children's diets. We also recommend old-fashioned hot oatmeal for breakfast. It cooks in 5 minutes. Just add warm 1% milk, cinnamon, and a small amount of non-caloric sweetener for another healthy breakfast choice.

Remember to add variety to meals. Some children are quite content to eat the same food every day at breakfast; others want more diversity. While there is a rule that breakfast must be eaten, there is no rule that only traditional breakfast foods should be served for the first meal of the day. Consider sandwiches of stone-ground wheat bread filled with lean ham and low-fat cheese. Add fillings to whole-wheat tortillas and pitas, or consider serving any other Sugar Busters favorite food.

Lunch, if a child eats it at school, can be a little more of a challenge to stay with the Sugar Busters plan. The National School Lunch Program is mandated to provide meals that "safeguard the health and well-being of the nation's children." Schools are required to provide lunches that meet the dietary guidelines for Americans. This includes a diet high in vegetables, fruits, and grains; 30% or less of calories from fat; and less than 10% of calories from saturated fat; it must also be moderate in sugar and salt. Lunches must also provide at least one-third of the daily Recommended Dietary Allowances for protein, iron, calcium, and vitamins A and C over the course of each school week.

We reviewed one city school district's lunch plan for the month of October 2000. The fat content was well within the limits of the dietary guidelines. But, unfortunately, since high-glycemic carbohydrates are not yet universally recognized for the negative effects of blood-sugar and insulin spikes that occur, almost all of the lunches were loaded with high-glycemic carbohydrates. We mean, simply, that starches were all too well represented. White potatoes, the most prevalent food, either french fried or mashed, appeared every other day. White rice, pizza, pasta, and "giant soft pretzels" were offered on other days. Hot dogs and sausage patties were served on buns. And we are quite sure the buns were not stone-ground, whole-wheat bread.

If it is too difficult to find the correct food choices at school, it may be necessary for your child to bring his or her own lunch from home, if the school will permit it. This will require a little planning and preparation on your part—and be sure to include your child in this endeavor. There are many alternatives to the traditional sandwich, since lunch bags are now equipped with air-tight containers and ice packs. If you prepare a salad, pack the low-fat dressing in a Ziploc bag. Add crunch to the greens with celery, sprouts, nuts, sunflower seeds, and broccoli florets. Don't discard those broccoli stems! Peel off the tough outer layer and serve them with a dip or slice them thin and add them to salads. The stems taste great and no one will know that it is broccoli.

Try whole-grain pita pockets stuffed with tuna or sliced chicken. Layer lean ham or turkey and low-fat cheese on a whole-wheat tortilla, add a favorite spread, and roll it up. Set aside some plain whole-wheat pasta from the night before and marinate it overnight with any combination of olive oil, green onions, garlic, spices, olives, red bell peppers, and raw vegetables for a school lunch that will be envied by your child's classmates.

If you are not using stone-ground wheat bread, now is the time to begin. You can introduce it in a "two-toned" sandwich, one slice of white and the other of wheat. Soon you will be able to substitute wheat for the white slice, and your children will wonder how they ever ate that mushy white bread that sticks to the roof of their mouths.

Dinner is family time, a meal that we recommend eating together as often as possible. We learned from the questionnaires that the Sugar

Busters way of eating is bringing family members together. Why not cook together too? There are countless reasons for family members to join in meal preparation, because cooking together cuts down on preparation time and gives mom and/or dad some help while they teach the Sugar Busters Way of Eating. It promotes team effort and co-operation and fosters independence. It helps teach math skills through measurements and conversions. It's economical, because take-out and eating out is expensive. And, most important, cooking together pro-motes conversation among family members.

Very often both parents are employed full time, and weeknights become frantic efforts to "get it all done." Carpooling, extracurricular activities, homework, and housework vie for the too-few hours left in the day. No wonder there is the great temptation to go to the drive-through and pick up that high-glycemic meal that brings the nagging guilt and broken promise to make a change . . . next week. Now is the time to enlist the help of the whole family. We recommend a Sugar Busters family meal-preparation time on weekends and week-days. On weekends, set aside one to two hours to meet in the kitchen to plan, wash, chop, Ziploc and Crock-Pot. On weeknights enlist family members to work as a team to cut down on last-minute prepara-tion time.

Planning: The Sugar Buster Pantry

Meal planning is essential in order to save time and resist the last-minute temptation to pick up fast food. Offer your family suggestions for Sugar Busters meals, and then let everyone take a turn choosing different menus. Keep a master list of ingredients for recipes, make copies, and check off items that you've run out of in order to facilitate grocery shopping. Choose from foods listed below to get you started on stocking a Sugar Busters pantry and refrigerator. The list is not exhaus-tive, but it will provide ingredients included in many of the recipes we offer. You can check the glycemic index tables for foods that you might want to serve but that do not appear on this list.

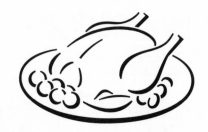

Meats

Canadian bacon	Lean ham (not sugar cured)
Lean turkey bacon	Lean pork
Lean ground beef	Quail and other game birds
Trimmed lean beef	Turkey
Chicken	Veal
Lamb	

Avoid fatty cuts of beef and lamb, sugar-cured ham and bacon, and cold cuts with sugar added.

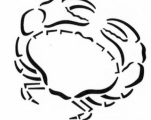

Seafood

Crab	Oysters
Crayfish	Bay and sea scallops
Fish of all kinds	Shrimp

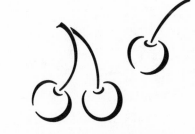

Fruit

Apples

Apricots

Berries

Cantaloupes

Cherries

Grapes

Honeydew melons

Kiwis

Lemons

Limes

Mangos

Nectarines

Oranges

Peaches

Pears

Plums

Tangerines

Avoid ripe bananas, pineapples, raisins, watermelon, frozen fruit with sugar added, and canned fruit in syrup.

THE SUGAR BUSTERS PANTRY

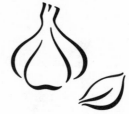

Vegetables

Artichokes	Garlic	Peas
Avocados	Ginger	Bell peppers
Dried beans of all kinds	Green beans	Chile peppers
Broccoli	Green onions	Spinach
Cabbage	Lentils	Squash
Cauliflower	Leeks	Sweet potatoes
Celery	Mushrooms	Greens
Cilantro	Okra	Tomatoes
Cucumbers	Onions	Zucchini
Eggplant	Parsley	Yams

Avoid beets, corn, parsnips, white potatoes (especially french fries), turnips, and frozen or canned vegetables with sugar added.

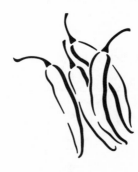

Dairy Products

Butter, in moderation

Cheese (preferably reduced fat)

Cottage cheese, low fat

Goat cheese

Eggs

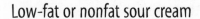

Egg substitute

Milk (skim or 1%)

Low-fat or nonfat sour cream

Yogurt with no sugar added (preferably low fat or nonfat)

Avoid yogurt made with sugar or maltodextrin added and
excessive consumption of high-fat dairy products.

THE SUGAR BUSTERS PANTRY

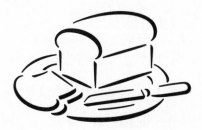

Baked Goods

Stone-ground whole-wheat bagels

Stone-ground whole-wheat breads

Whole-grain breads

Stone-ground whole-wheat crackers

Whole-wheat tortillas

Bran or stone-ground whole-grain muffins sweetened with fruit juice, fructose, or artificial sweeteners

Avoid breads made with refined, enriched, or bleached flour; breads that have added honey, molasses, corn syrup, or brown sugar; breads that have more than one gram of sugar per slice; and most pastries, which are not only high in sugar but high in fat.

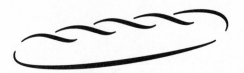

Canned Goods, Condiments, Etc.

Artichoke bottoms
and hearts

Beans

Beef broth
(reduced sodium)

Chicken broth
(reduced sodium)

Green chiles

Hearts of palm

Prepared horseradish

Ketchup, in moderation

Reduced-fat mayonnaise

Mustards

Nuts (dry roasted)

Canola oil

Olive oil

Oil sprays

Olives

Plain and pickled
jalapeño peppers

Roasted red peppers

Salsas

Hot sauce

Reduced-sodium soy
sauce

Worcestershire sauce

No-sugar-added
spreadable fruit

Tomato juice

Tomato purée

No-sugar-added
tomato sauce

Tomatoes

Tuna

Balsamic vinegar

Cider vinegar

White vinegar

Red wine vinegar

Avoid baked beans, sweet pickles, sugar-sweetened jams, jellies,
and preserves, salad dressings with sugar added.

THE SUGAR BUSTERS PANTRY

97

Dry Packaged Products

High-bran cereals with no sugar added

Whole-grain cereals with no sugar added

Whole-grain crackers

Whole-wheat croutons

Stone-ground whole-wheat flour

Artificial sweeteners

Splenda

Whole, rolled, or steel-cut oats

Whole-wheat pastas

Stone-ground pitas

Brown rice (not instant)

Basmati rice

Whole-wheat tortillas

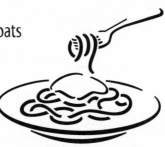

Avoid cold cereals with sugar added, Cream of Wheat, flavored instant hot cereals, regular crackers, all-purpose and other enriched flour, products made with enriched flour, sugar, significant amounts of white pastas, white rice, and risotto.

Preparation

Now that you have done your grocery shopping, checking labels and making sure that you have made the correct Sugar Busters choices, it is time to gather the family together for food preparation that will make weeknight cooking less of a hassle. Don't forget the necessary plastic containers and Ziploc and freezer bags that will be essential for food storage. Here are some ideas for preparation and cooking ahead that will cut down on time later. Recipes using many of the ideas will follow.

○ Dig deep into your kitchen cabinet and dust off the once popular Crock-Pot. Vegetables retain their natural juices from the moist cooking, and lean but tough cuts of meat become tenderized. Add all ingredients to the slow cooker at once, cut liquids by half in most recipes, and return hours later to a nutritious and flavorful meal. No need to worry about burning or overcooking food, and no need to add flour to create a flavorful gravy. Crock-Pots are perfect for cooking soups, stews, and also beans, chicken, and roasts.

○ Wash, trim, and slice vegetables and greens. Weekday meal preparation is easy if you have bags of sliced onions, celery, garlic, bell peppers, and mushrooms ready to add to a casserole, skillet, stir-fry, grilled, or baked dish. Salads are easy to prepare when the greens are already washed, dried, refrigerated, and crisp. Other vegetables can be sliced or chopped and stored. It is better to wash them just before meal preparation to preserve freshness.

○ If stone-ground wheat breadcrumbs are not available in your area, make your own. Break up slices of wheat bread into the bowl of your food processor, process until fine, toast on a baking sheet in the oven, cool completely, and store in airtight bags in the refrigerator.

○ Use a hamburger press to cut round slices out of stone-ground wheat bread for mini pizzas or snack foods. Use your food processor to make breadcrumbs with the left-over crusts.

O Grill, broil, or bake skinless, seasoned chicken filets. Slice chicken into thin strips to use later in fajitas, pita pockets, or to top salads. Keeping grilled, broiled, or baked chicken on hand is a great time saver for quick meal preparation.

O Boil wheat pasta ahead and add olive oil after cooking to prevent sticking. Refrigerate this and use it during the week as salads, or reheat it and add a quick stir-fry topping.

O Make your own oven-baked, whole-wheat tortilla chips for snacks. Cut refrigerated wheat tortillas into wedges and toast lightly under the broiler.

O Chicken, beef, and vegetable stocks can be easily prepared, left to simmer for hours, cooled, refrigerated, and frozen to later become the base for soups and casseroles. Fat is easy to skim off of the top of chilled stock.

A Few of Our Favorite Foods

Tomatoes: Research indicates that populations with a regular consumption of tomato products have a lower incidence of cardiovascular disease and nutritionally linked cancers. Cooking seems to release important antioxidants in tomatoes (Weisburger). Is there any more versatile fruit? Look for low- or no-sugar-added canned tomatoes. Some brands include spices that provide great flavor when added to bean, soup, and vegetable dishes. Don't forget homemade fresh salsas prepared with fresh tomatoes, garlic, and cilantro as a delicious and nutritious dip or topping for salads.

Lentils: One Sugar Buster author plugs lentils as "the perfect carbohydrate"! With a glycemic index of 29, second only to soybeans as a usable source of protein, containing no cholesterol and virtually no fat, lentils may very well be just that. This legume, which is one of the oldest known food crops (originating around 7000 B.C.), can be used in soups, stews, and salad dishes.

Basmati rice: It is mild in flavor, cooks quickly, and has a low glycemic index of 58. Basmati rice is a great alternative to brown rice. Add stir-fry vegetables, light turkey sausage, and spice for a meal in one pot.

Beans: Black, red, white—in any color, they can be eaten alone or added to soups, casseroles, salads for extra fiber. Dried beans can be simmered for hours with spices and lean ham for seasoning. When they are tender, a small amount can be removed and mashed, then returned to the pot to thicken gravy, avoiding the use of flour. Canned black beans, rinsed and drained, are included in many new recipes. Combined with other ingredients, they will be less noticeable to kids who may balk at the idea of eating beans. They offer the same fiber benefits as dried beans and are less time-consuming to prepare.

Fruits: For maximum benefits, most fruit should be eaten with the skin on. Consider adding **mangos** and **kiwifruit** to your fruit basket. Mangos are good sources of fiber and make wonderful fruit salsas. One kiwifruit contains all of the recommended daily vitamin C.

Soy: Soy has been part of the Southeast Asian diet for nearly five millennia and is rapidly gaining attention for use in the Western diet because it is a superior source of plant protein, it has protein quality equal to that of meat, and it has the potential to decrease the risk of some cancers and cardiovascular disease. The United States Food and Drug Administration recently approved the health claim for soy's role in reducing the risk of cardiovascular disease. Consider substituting tofu for meat in some of your recipes to reduce the amount of calories, fat, and cholesterol that beef will add. Soy is cholesterol free.

Tea: Tea is the second most highly consumed beverage in the world and has been popular for over 4,000 years. Green and black teas have the richest source of antioxidants, called flavonoids. Tea also contains vitamins and fluoride. Research is showing that moderate amounts of tea may protect against several forms of cancer, cardiovascular diseases, formation of kidney stones, bacterial infections, and dental cavities.

Fish: Grilled, baked, broiled, or poached fish is quick and easy to prepare. More and more studies are showing that the omega-3 fatty acids (healthy fat) found in fish oils provide protection against heart disease. One to two 3-ounce servings of fish rich in omega-3s every week is recommended. Salmon, anchovies, albacore, bluefin tuna, and sardines are the richest sources of omega-3 fatty acids.

16

Meal Plans

The Sugar Busters food pyramid and suggested meal plans are guides that will be helpful for an easy transition to the Sugar Busters lifestyle. They have been designed to provide a variety of foods for a healthy way of eating. Remember, by introducing your family to a variety of foods, even those they may not be accustomed to eating, and repeatedly offering these foods, you are providing them with many opportunities to consume the nutrients and make the food choices necessary for disease prevention and healthy weight.

Food Pyramid

A food pyramid is a pictorial representation of the recommended daily intake of items from each food group. The Sugar Busters food pyramid is designed to reflect the Sugar Busters concept and is a modification of the USDA food pyramid. The Sugar Busters pyramid includes all the food groups and is a guide to help you choose a variety of foods that contain the vital nutrients you need and that are necessary for maintaining a healthy weight. One difference between the USDA and the Sugar Busters pyramid is that we emphasize the consumption of high-fiber, whole-grain foods. The Sugar Busters pyramid has a separate

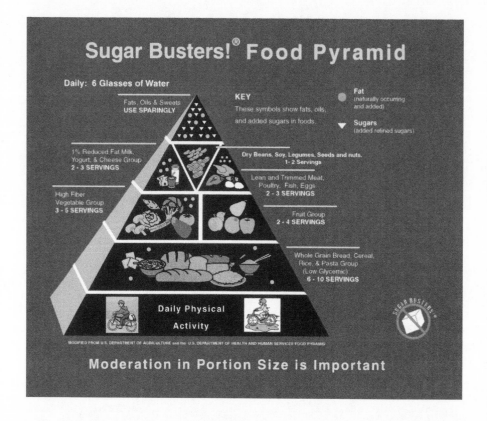

Sugar Busters!® Food Pyramid

Daily: 6 Glasses of Water

Fats, Oils & Sweets
USE SPARINGLY

KEY
These symbols show fats, oils,
and added sugars in foods.

Fat
(naturally occurring
and added)

Sugars
(added refined sugars)

1% Reduced Fat Milk,
Yogurt, & Cheese Group
2 - 3 SERVINGS

Dry Beans, Soy, Legumes, Seeds and nuts.
1- 2 Servings

Lean and Trimmed Meat,
Poultry, Fish, Eggs
2 - 3 SERVINGS

High Fiber
Vegetable Group
3 - 5 SERVINGS

Fruit Group
2 - 4 SERVINGS

Whole Grain Bread, Cereal,
Rice, & Pasta Group
(Low Glycemic)
6 - 10 SERVINGS

Daily Physical
Activity

MODIFIED FROM U.S. DEPARTMENT OF AGRICULTURE and the U.S. DEPARTMENT OF HEALTH AND HUMAN SERVICES FOOD PYRAMID

Moderation in Portion Size is Important

category for beans and legumes, indicating the importance we give these foods. Other differences are that we recommend 1% reduced-fat milk and we encourage daily exercise. The small area at the top of the pyramid signifies the importance of limiting added sugars and fats.

The two seven-day meal plans that follow have been designed to meet the nutritional needs of six- to eight-year-olds and nine- to twelve-year-olds. The plans are intended as guides and can be adapted to the preferences of your children. The daily meals can be consumed in any order and substitutions within a food group are encouraged. (For example, a child may prefer wheat pasta instead of brown rice.) Since most recipes in current books and magazines give the macro-nutrient values of the ingredients, substitution becomes an easy matter. Conversely, your child may not want variety and choose peanut butter and jelly on whole-wheat bread for lunch several days in a row. Or your child may want the same breakfast food each day, which is acceptable, with the exception of a daily egg breakfast. It is very important to try to make every effort to offer at least the minimum servings from each food group on a daily basis.

Remember to consider the glycemic load theory when creating a meal. Don't overdose on carbohydrates. The amount of carbohydrates we recommend each day is 200 grams to 225 grams for the six- to eight-year-old group and 240 grams to 260 grams for the nine- to twelve-year-old group.

The asterisks in the meal plan indicate that a recipe for the food can be found in the recipe section of this book.

Menu for Child 6 to 8 Years Old

Day 1	Portion Size	Food	Exchanges	g Carbohydrates
Breakfast	1/2 cup	Shredded wheat	1 starch	15
	1 cup (8 fl. oz.)	1% milk	1 milk	12
	1/2 cup	Fresh strawberries	1 fruit	5
	1 slice (1 oz.)	Whole-wheat toast	1 starch	15
	1 tsp.	Margarine	1 fat	0
	2 tsp.	Spreadable Fruit (Polaner®)	free	6
				53
Snack	1 cup	Green tea	free	0
	1/2 cup (4 oz.)	Lowfat, no-sugar-added vanilla yogurt	1/2 milk	6
				6
Lunch	Ham and cheese sandwich on pumpernickel			
	2 slices	Pumpernickel bread	2 starches	30
	1 slice (1 oz.)	Ham	1 meat	0
	1 slice (1 oz.)	Provolone cheese	1 meat sub.	0
	1 tsp.	Mustard	free	0
	1 cup	Salad, mixed greens	1 vegetable	0
	9 nuts	Almonds or cashews	1 1/2 fats	0
	2 tbsp.	Ranch Dressing (Sugar Busters!®)	1 1/2 fats	0
	1 cup (8 fl. oz.)	1% milk	1 milk	12
				42
Snack	17 small	Fresh grapes	1 fruit	15
	1/2 cup (4 fl. oz.)	1% milk	1/2 milk	6
				21
Dinner	1/2 cup	Quick Red Beans (kidney)*	1 starch, 1 meat	15
	1/2 cup	Brown rice, cooked	1 1/2 starches	22
	1 oz.	Ham	1 meat	0
	1 cup	Spinach	2 vegetables	2
	2 tsp.	Margarine	2 fats	0
	1 cup	Grape juice	2 fruits	30
				69
			Daily total	191

Menu for Child 6 to 8 Years Old

Day 2	Portion Size	Food	Exchanges	g Carbohydrates
Breakfast	1/2 cup	Apple Cinnamon Oatmeal*	1 starch	19
	1 cup	1% milk	1 milk	12
	1 slice (1 oz.)	Whole-wheat toast	1 starch	15
	1 tsp.	Margarine	1 fat	0
				46
Snack	6	Whole-wheat crackers	1 starch	15
	1/2 cup	1% milk	1/2 milk	6
				21
Lunch	Tuna salad Sandwich			
	2 oz.	Tuna, packed in water (drained)	2 meats	0
	2 slices (2 oz.)	Rye bread	2 starches	30
	2 tbsp.	Mayonnaise, sugar-free	2 fats	0
	1 leaf	Romaine lettuce	free	0
	1/4 cup	Tomato, sliced	1/4 vegetable	0
	1 cup	Salad greens	1 vegetable	0
	1 tbsp.	Salad dressing	1 fat	0
	1 cup	1% milk	1 milk	12
				42
Snack	2	Fresh plums	1 fruit	15
	1/2 cup	1% milk	1/2 milk	6
				21
Dinner	Meat Sauce and Pasta*			
	1/2 cup	Meat sauce	1 starch, 1 fat	15
	1/2 cup	Whole-wheat angel hair pasta	1 1/2 starches	28
	1/2 cup	Green peas, canned	2 vegetables	11
	1 tsp.	Margarine	1 fat	0
	2/3 cup	Cranberry juice	2 fruits	30
				84
			Daily total	214

Menu for Child 6 to 8 Years Old

Day 3	Portion Size	Food	Exchanges	g Carbohydrates
Breakfast	1/2 (2 oz.)	Bagel, whole wheat	2 starches	30
	1 tbsp.	Cream cheese	2 fats	0
	1/2 cup	1% milk	1/2 milk	6
				36
Snack	1/2 cup	Homemade Trail Mix*	1 starch,	22
			1/2 fat, 1/2 fruit	
	1/2 cup	1% milk	1/2 milk	6
				28
Lunch		Grilled cheese sandwich		
	2 slices (2 oz.)	Whole-wheat bread	2 starches	30
	2 slices (2 oz.)	American cheese	2 meat sub.	0
	1 tsp.	Margarine	1 fat	0
		Fresh salad with homemade dressing		
	1 cup	Fresh baby greens	1 vegetable	0
	1/2 cup	Fresh cucumbers &	1/2 vegetable	0
		tomatoes, sliced		
	1/2 tbsp.	Red wine vinegar	free	0
	1/2 tbsp.	Balsamic vinegar	free	0
	1 tsp.	Olive oil	1 fat	0
	2 tsp.	Mustard	free	0
	1/2 cup	Fresh blueberries	1/2 fruit	10
	1 cup	1% milk	1 milk	12
				52
Snack	1 oz.	Whole-Wheat Pita Triangles*	1 starch	15
	1/4 cup	Tomato Salsa*	1/2 vegetable	3
	1/2 cup	1% milk	1/2 milk	6
				24
Dinner	2 oz.	Grilled Chicken Breast*	2 meats	0
	1/2 cup	Sweet Potato Frisbees*	1 starch	15
	1/2 cup	Spicy Lentils*	1 1/2 vegetables	20
	1/2 (1/2 oz.)	Whole-wheat roll	1/2 starch	7
	1 tsp.	Margarine	1 fat	0
	1/2 cup	Apple juice	1 fruit	15
				57
			Daily total	197

Menu for Child 6 to 8 Years Old

Day 4	Portion Size	Food	Exchanges	g Carbohydrates
Breakfast	2 each (4.5 in. across)	Whole-wheat waffles, toasted	2 starches, 2 fats	30
	2 tbsp.	Syrup, sugar free	free	0
	2 tsp.	Margarine	2 fats	0
	1 cup	Fresh strawberries, sliced	1 fruit	10
	1 cup	1% milk	1 milk	12
				52
Snack	4	Triscuits®	1 starch	13
	1/2 cup	Apple juice	1 fruit	15
				28
Lunch	Bean Burritos*			
	2 each (6 in. across)	Tortillas (whole wheat)	2 starches	30
	1/2 cup	Black beans, canned	1 starch, 1 meat sub.	17
	1/2 cup (2 oz.)	Monterey Jack cheese	2 meat sub.	0
	1/4 cup	Salsa	free	0
	1/2 cup	Fresh tomatoes, diced	1/2 vegetable	4
	1/2 cup	Zucchini Stir Fry*	1 vegetable	10
	1/2 cup	1% milk	1/2 milk	6
				67
Snack	12 each	Fresh cherries	1 fruit	15
	1/2 cup	1% milk	1/2 milk	6
				21
Dinner	Broccoli Pasta Soup*		see recipe	
	1 cup	Broccoli Soup		25
	Bagel Pizza*			
	1/2 (1 oz.)	Whole-wheat bagel	1 starch	15
	2 tbsp.	Marinara sauce	free	0
	1/4 cup (1 oz.)	Mozzarella, shredded	1 meat sub.	2
	1/2 cup	Fresh mushrooms, sliced	1/2 vegetable	2
	1 cup	1% milk	1 milk	12
				56
			Daily total	224

6 TO 8 YEARS OLD

Menu for Child 6 to 8 Years Old

Day 5	Portion Size	Food	Exchanges	g Carbohydrates
Breakfast	1 each (4 in. across)	Whole-Wheat Buttermilk Pancakes*	see recipe	16
	2 tbsp.	Syrup, sugar free	free	0
	3/4 cup	Fresh blueberries, whole or puréed	1 fruit	15
	1 cup	1% milk	1 milk	12
				43
Snack	Pinwheel*			
	1 slice (1 oz.)	Whole-wheat bread, no ends	1 starch	15
	1 tsp.	Spreadable fruit (Polaner®)	free	3
	1/2 cup	1% milk	1/2 milk	6
				24
Lunch	Turkey sandwich			
	2 slices (2 oz.)	Rye bread	2 starches	30
	2 oz.	Turkey breast	2 meats	0
	1 tsp.	Brown mustard	free	0
	1 cup	Fresh zucchini sticks	1 vegetable	0
	1 tbsp.	Ranch dressing	1 fat	0
	1/2 cup	Orange juice	1 fruit	15
				45
Snack	1/2 cup (4 oz.)	Yogurt, lowfat, no sugar added	1/2 milk	6
	1/2 cup	Apple juice	1 fruit	15
				21
Dinner	Chicken Fusilli Pasta*		see recipe	48
	1/2 cup	Green Beans and Onions*	1 vegetable	4
	1 tsp.	Margarine	1 fat	0
	1 cup	1% milk	1 milk	12
				64
			Daily total	197

Menu for Child 6 to 8 Years Old

Day 6	Portion Size	Food	Exchanges	g Carbohydrates
Breakfast	Cheese and Tomato Omelet*		see recipe	5
	1 slice	Whole-wheat bread	1 starch	15
	1 tsp.	Margarine	1 fat	0
	1/2 cup	Orange juice	1 fruit	15
				35
Snack	1 fruit	Apple	1 fruit	21
	1/2 cup	1% milk	1 milk	6
				27
Lunch	Peanut butter & jelly sandwich			
	2 slices (2 oz.)	Whole-wheat bread	2 starches	30
	2 tbsp.	Peanut butter	1 meat substitute	6
	1 tbsp.	Spreadable fruit	1 fruit	10
	1/2 cup	Fresh celery sticks, sliced	1/2 vegetable	0
	1 tbsp.	Ranch dressing	1 fat	0
	1 cup	1% milk	1 milk	12
				58
Snack	Sugar Busters®	Sugar Busters! Ice Cream	2 milk	24
	Ice Cream Float*	or no-sugar-added ice cream		
				24
Dinner	Basmati Rice Jambalaya*		see recipe	41
	1/2 cup	Broccoli, steamed	1 vegetable	2
	2 tsp.	Margarine	2 fats	0
	1/2 cup	1% milk	1 milk	6
				49
			Daily total	193

6 TO 8 YEARS OLD

Menu for Child 6 to 8 Years Old

Day 7	Portion Size	Food	Exchanges	g Carbohydrates
Breakast	1/2 cup	Whole-grain cereal	1 starch	15
	1 slice	Whole-wheat toast	1 starch	15
	1 tbsp.	Spreadable fruit	1 fruit	10
	2 tsp.	Margarine	2 fats	0
	1 slice	Canadian bacon	1 meat	0
	1 cup	1% milk	1 milk	12
				52
Snack	Fruit Squiggles*			
	1/2 cup	Sugar-free gelatin	1 fruit	15
		(prepared with apple juice)		
	1 cup	Green tea	free	0
				15
Lunch	Quesadillas*		see recipe	
	1 each (6 in. across)			15
	1/2 cup	Pinto beans	1 starch,	22
			1 meat sub.	
	3/4 cup	Zucchini, steamed	1 1/2 vegetables	5
	1 tsp.	Margarine	1 fat	0
	1 cup	1% milk	1 milk	12
				54
Snack	1/2 cup	Vanilla pudding, sugar free	1 starch	15
		(made with lowfat milk)		
	1/2 cup	1% milk	1 milk	6
				21
Dinner	Taco Salad*		see recipe	9
	1/2 pita	Whole-wheat pita pocket	1 starch	17
	3/4 cup	Sweet Potato Frisbees*	1 1/2 starches	22
	1/2 cup	Orange juice	1 fruit	15
				63
			Daily total	205

Menu for Child 9 to 12 Years Old

Day 1	Portion Size	Food	Exchanges	g Carbohydrates
Breakfast	1/2 cup	Shredded wheat	1 starch	15
	1 cup (8 fl. oz.)	1% milk	1 milk	12
	1/2 cup	Fresh strawberries	1 fruit	5
	1 slice (1 oz.)	Whole-wheat toast	1 starch	15
	1 tsp.	Margarine	1 fat	0
	2 tsp.	Spreadable Fruit (Polaner®)	free	6
				53
Snack	1 cup	Green tea	free	0
	1 cup (8 fl. oz.)	Lowfat, no-sugar-added vanilla yogurt	1 milk	12
				12
Lunch	Ham and cheese sandwich on pumpernickel			
	2 slices	Pumpernickel bread	2 starches	30
	2 slices (2 oz.)	Ham	2 meats	0
	1 slice (1 oz.)	Provolone cheese	1 meat sub.	0
	1 tsp.	Mustard	free	0
	1 cup	Salad, mixed greens	1 vegetable	0
	9	Almonds or cashews	1 1/2 fats	0
	2 tbsp.	Ranch dressing (Sugar Busters!®)	2 fats	0
	1 cup (8 fl. oz.)	1% milk	1 milk	12
				42
Snack	17 small	Fresh grapes	1 fruit	15
	1 cup (8 fl. oz.)	1% milk	1 milk	12
				27
Dinner	1/2 cup	Quick Red Beans (kidney)*	1 starch, 1 meat	15
	1 cup	Brown rice, cooked	3 starches	45
	1 oz.	Ham	1 meat	0
	1 cup	Spinach	2 vegetables	2
	2 tsp.	Margarine	2 fats	0
	1 (1 oz.)	Whole-wheat roll	1 starch	15
	1 cup	Grape juice	2 fruits	30
			Daily total	107
				241

9 TO 12 YEARS OLD

Menu for Child 9 to 12 Years Old

Day 2	Portion Size	Food	Exchanges	g Carbohydrates
Breakfast	1 cup	Apple Cinnamon Oatmeal*	1 1/2 starches	38
	1 cup	1% milk	1 milk	12
	1 slice (1 oz.)	Whole-wheat toast	1 starch	15
	1 tsp.	Margarine	1 fat	0
				65
Snack	6	Whole-wheat crackers	1 starch	15
	1 oz.	Mozzarella cheese	1 lean meat, 1 fat	1
	1 cup	1% milk	1 milk	12
				28
Lunch	Tuna salad sandwich			
	2 oz.	Tuna, packed in water (drained)	2 meats	0
	2 slices (2 oz.)	Rye	2 starches	30
	2 tbsp.	Mayonnaise, lowfat	2 fats	0
	1 leaf	Romaine lettuce	free	0
	1/4 cup	Tomato, sliced	1/4 vegetable	0
	1 cup	Fresh salad greens	1 vegetable	0
	1 tbsp.	Salad dressing	1 fat	0
	1 cup	1% milk	1 milk	12
				42
Snack	2	Fresh plums	1 fruit	15
	1/2 cup	1% milk	1/2 milk	6
				21
Dinner	Meat Sauce and Pasta*		see recipe	57
	1 cup	Meat sauce		
	1 cup	Whole-wheat angel hair pasta		
	1/2 cup	Green peas, canned	2 vegetables	11
	1 tsp.	Margarine	1 fat	0
	1 cup	Cranberry juice	2 fruits	30
				98
			Daily total	254

Menu for Child 9 to 12 Years Old

Day 3	Portion Size	Food	Exchanges	g Carbohydrates
Breakfast	1 (2 oz.)	Bagel, whole wheat	2 starches	30
	2 tbsp.	Cream cheese	2 fats	0
	1 cup	1% milk	1 milk	12
				42
Snack	1/2 cup	Homemade Trail Mix*	1 starch,	22
			1/2 fat, 1/2 fruit	
	1/2 cup	1% milk	1 milk	6
				28
Lunch	Grilled cheese sandwich			
	2 slices (2 oz.)	Whole-wheat bread	2 starches	30
	2 slices (2 oz.)	American cheese	2 meat sub.	0
	2 tsp.	Margarine	2 fats	0
	Fresh salad with homemade dressing			
	1 cup	Fresh baby greens	1 vegetable	0
	1/2 cup	Fresh cucumbers & tomatoes, sliced	1/2 vegetable	0
	1/2 tbsp.	Red wine vinegar	free	0
	1/2 tbsp.	Balsamic vinegar	free	0
	1 tsp.	Olive oil	1 fat	0
	2 tsp.	Mustard	free	0
	3/4 cup	Fresh blueberries	1 fruit	15
	1 cup	1% milk	1 milk	12
				57
Snack	1 oz.	Whole-Wheat Pita Triangles*	1 starch	15
	1/4 cup	Tomata Salsa*	1/2 vegetable	3
	1/2 cup	1% milk	1/2 milk	6
				24
Dinner	3 oz.	Grilled Chicken Breast*	3 meats	0
	1 cup	Sweet Potato Frisbees*	2 starches	30
	1/2 cup	Spicy Lentils*	1 1/2 vegetables	20
	1 (1 oz.)	Whole-wheat roll	1 starch	15
	1 tsp.	Margarine	1 fat	0
	1 cup	Apple juice	2 fruits	30
				95
			Daily total	246

9 TO 12 YEARS OLD

115

Menu for Child 9 to 12 Years Old

Day 4	Portion Size	Food	Exchanges	g Carbohydrates
Breakfast	2 each (4.5 in. across)	Whole-wheat waffles, toasted	2 starches, 2 fats	30
	2 tbsp.	Syrup, sugar free	free	0
	2 tsp.	Margarine	2 fats	0
	1 cup	Fresh strawberries, sliced	1 fruit	10
	1 cup	1% milk	1 milk	12
				52
Snack	7	Triscuits®	1 1/2 starches, 1 fat	22
	1/2 cup	Apple juice	1 fruit	15
				37
Lunch	Bean Burritos*			
	2 each (6 in. across)	Tortillas (whole wheat)	2 starches	30
	1/2 cup	Black beans, canned	1/2 starch, 1/2 meat sub.	17
	1/2 cup (2 oz.)	Monterey Jack cheese	2 meat sub.	0
	2 tbsp.	Sour cream	1 fat	0
	1/4 cup	Salsa	free	0
	1/2 cup	Fresh tomatoes, diced	1/2 vegetable	4
	1/2 cup	Zucchini Stir Fry*	1 vegetable	10
	1 cup	1% milk	1 milk	12
				73
Snack	12	Fresh cherries	1 fruit	15
	1 cup	1% milk	1 milk	12
				27
Dinner	Broccoli Pasta Soup*		see recipe	
	1 cup	Broccoli Soup		25
	Bagel Pizza*			
	1/2 (1 oz.)	Whole-wheat bagel	1 starch	15
	2 tbsp.	Marinara sauce	free	0
	2 oz.	Mozzarella, shredded	2 meat sub.	0
	1/2 cup	Fresh mushrooms, sliced	1/2 vegetable	2
	1 cup	1% milk	1 milk	12
				54
			Daily total	243

9 TO 12 YEARS OLD

116

Menu for Child 9 to 12 Years Old

Day 5	Portion Size	Food	Exchanges	g Carbohydrates
Breakfast	2 each (4 in. across)	Whole-Wheat Buttermilk Pancakes*	2 starch, 1 fat	33
	2 tbsp.	Syrup, sugar free	free	0
	3/4 cup	Fresh blueberries, whole	1 fruit	15
	1 cup	1% milk	1 milk	12
				60
Snack	Pinwheel*			
	1 slice (1 oz.)	Whole-wheat bread, no ends	1 starch	15
	1 tsp.	Spreadable fruit (Polaner®)	free	3
	1 cup	1% milk	1 milk	12
				30
Lunch	Turkey sandwich			
	2 slices (2 oz.)	Rye bread	2 starches	30
	2 oz.	Turkey breast	2 meats	0
	1 tsp.	Brown mustard	free	0
	1 cup	Fresh zucchini sticks	1 vegetable	0
	1 tbsp.	Ranch dressing	1 fat	0
	1/2 cup	Orange juice	1 fruit	15
				45
Snack	1 cup (8 oz.)	Yogurt, lowfat, no sugar added	1 milk	12
	1/2 cup	Apple juice	1 fruit	15
				27
Dinner	Chicken Fusilli Pasta*		see recipe	48
	1 cup	Green Beans and Onions*	2 vegetables	8
	2 tsp.	Margarine	2 fats	0
	1 cup	1% milk	1 milk	12
				68
			Daily total	230

9 TO 12 YEARS OLD

Menu for Child 9 to 12 Years Old

Day 6	Portion Size	Food	Exchanges	g Carbohydrates
Breakfast	Cheese and Tomato Omelet*		see recipe	5
	2 slices	Whole-wheat bread	2 starches	30
	1 tsp.	Margarine	1 fat	0
	1 cup	Orange juice	2 fruit	30
				65
Snack	1 fruit	Apple	1 fruit	21
	1 cup	1% milk	1 milk	12
				33
Lunch	Peanut butter & jelly sandwich			
	2 slices (2 oz.)	Whole-wheat bread	2 starches	30
	2 tbsp.	Peanut butter	1 meat sub.	6
	1 tbsp.	Spreadable fruit	1 fruit	10
	1/2 cup	Fresh celery sticks, sliced	1/2 vegetable	0
	1 tbsp.	Ranch dressing	1 fat	0
	1 cup	1% milk	1 milk	12
				58
Snack	SugarBusters!® Ice Cream Float*	Sugar Busters! Ice Cream or no-sugar-added ice cream	2 milks	24
				24
Dinner	Basmati Rice Jambalaya*		see recipe	41
	1/2 cup	Broccoli, steamed	1 vegetable	2
	2 tsp.	Margarine	2 fats	0
	1 cup	1% milk	1 milk	12
				55
			Daily total	235

9 TO 12 YEARS OLD

Menu for Child 9 to 12 Years Old

Day 7	Portion Size	Food	Exchanges	g Carbohydrates
Breakfast	1/2 cup	Whole-grain cereal	1 starch	15
	1 slice	Whole-wheat toast	1 starch	15
	1 tbsp.	Spreadable fruit	1 fruit	10
	2 tsp.	Margarine	2 fats	0
	1 slice (1 oz.)	Canadian bacon	1 meat	0
	1 cup	1% milk	1 milk	12
				52
Snack	Fruit Squiggles*			
	1/2 cup	Sugar-free gelatin (prepared with apple juice)	1 fruit	15
	1 cup	Green tea	free	0
				15
Lunch	Quesadillas*		see recipe	
	2 each (6 in. across)			30
	1/2 cup	Pinto beans	1 starch, 1 meat sub.	22
	3/4 cup	Zucchini, steamed	11/2 vegetables	5
	1 tsp.	Butter	1 fat	0
	1 cup	1% milk	1 milk	12
				69
Snack	5	Triscuits®	1 starch, 1 fat	15
	1 cup	1% milk	1 milk	12
				27
Dinner	Taco Salad*		see recipe	9
	1/2 pita	Whole-wheat pita pocket	1 starch	17
	1 cup	Sweet Potato Frisbees*	2 starches	30
	1 cup	Orange juice	2 fruits	30
				86
			Daily total	249

9 TO 12 YEARS OLD

17

Recipes

The foods discussed in this book are the basis for planning and creating a nutritious way of eating. Now you can use these recommended foods as ingredients in the following recipes and find that they are every bit as tasty as the sugar-laden, greasy, high-glycemic fast foods you and your children may be accustomed to eating. We rarely hear that anyone has difficulty creating and maintaining a Sugar Busters eating plan for the entire family. With the suggestions, meal plans, and recipes in *Sugar Busters! Cut Sugar to Trim Fat*, *Sugar Busters! Quick and Easy Cookbook*, and now *Sugar Busters! for Kids*, incorporating the Sugar Busters lifestyle into lifelong healthy eating patterns can be a simple matter.

There is no better way of eating than quick, simply prepared, low-glycemic fresh fruits, vegetables, lean meats, chicken, seafood, and whole grains. However, everyone wants and needs variety. The recipes in this section will introduce you to the preparation of various foods discussed in this book that may be less familiar to people living in the Western world, and will assist in your efforts to avoid the routine American diet of refined sugar, meat, white potatoes, and fast food.

Let us consider a practical and healthy way of teaming different foods in a meal. Choose an entrée that requires some time to complete and pair it with a simply prepared steamed vegetable or salad. Or grill, broil, or bake an entrée of fish, lean meat, or skinless chicken and serve it with a more involved vegetable casserole or bean dish. To save time, look for variations following many of the recipes that add ingredients allowing you to create a one-dish meal. Don't overload on carbohydrates! For example, if you prepare a pasta, rice, sweet potato, or stuffing dish, avoid serving bread at the same meal.

These low-glycemic, high-fiber recipes will take you on a gastronomic journey around the world and offer a whole new experience of eating healthy, nutritious foods common in other cultures. Sugar Busters recommends the best foods chosen from other cuisines to add exciting tastes to your diet and variety to your meal plan. Try the lentils and basmati rice from India and the Middle East, soybeans (tofu) from Asia, black beans from Mexico and the Caribbean. Prepare recipes with chickpeas, olive oil, tomatoes, and wheat pasta from the Mediterranean region and bulgur from the Middle East. Eat the dense multigrain breads common in northern Europe, mangos from the tropics, and kiwis from New Zealand. Look to the United States for green beans, sweet potatoes, blueberries, greens, and seafood. These are just a few of the many possibilities for adding diversity to your way of eating.

While it is easy to find an abundance of food choices in many cultures, conversely there are many foods to be avoided in the same cultures. Avoid the corn and white-flour tortillas of Hispanic cuisines; the white potatoes of Irish, Hungarian, and Russian stews; the white rice, white breads, and highly processed grains of the United States. Does this mean that you have to give up an entire regional cuisine such as Creole or Cajun cooking? Absolutely not! Creole and Cajun dishes are known both for their spiciness and for the thick rouxs made from browning white flour in fat, such as butter or oil. Substitute stone-ground wheat flour for the white flour in the preparation of the roux, use less flour and less oil, add the wonderful spices, and you create Sugar Busters Creole, every bit as delicious, but oh so much healthier.

You will notice that the recipes with a higher fat content contain olive oil or canola oil as an ingredient. These oils are monounsaturated fats, which, in moderation, are considered healthy fats. We have limited the use of ingredients that are high in fat. Broiling, baking, grilling, sautéing, roasting, steaming, and simmering are all methods of cooking that are recommended instead of frying because frying increases the fat content of the food. Choose liquid vegetable oils that are high in unsaturated fats: canola, olive, peanut, safflower, sesame, soybean, and sunflower oils.

Select fresh or dried spices to add flavor to foods instead of cooking with saturated oils or preparing heavy flour sauces. At first glance some of the recipes may seem to have a large number of ingredients. Look carefully and you will find that many of the ingredients are spices, easy to stock up on and quick to add, resulting in flavorful dishes without excessive amounts of sugar and fat.

Our recipes are moderate in sodium content. Although the maximum recommended amount of salt or sodium for one day has not been established, the USDA suggests a daily value of 2,400 mg. of sodium for a moderate intake. This is equal to one teaspoon of salt. Salt is found mainly in processed and commercially prepared foods. This highlights the importance of careful reading of labels and brand comparison. Low-sodium canned broth, soy sauce, tomato products, or even better, fresh vegetables, can be used to reduce the sodium content of many recipes.

Until recently, some of the ingredients in the recipes were found only in specialty food stores. Today, fresh cilantro, mangos and kiwis, bulgur, brown rice, basmati rice, tofu, and whole-grain, whole-wheat breads and cereals are easily found in supermarkets. So join the ranks of consumers who are demanding and buying nutritious foods for their families. Stock your pantry with the correct foods; take the time to prepare these recipes; enjoy the variety of flavors and benefit from a healthier way of eating.

Breakfast

Breakfast Casserole with Eggs and Canadian Bacon

Servings: 4

A weekend treat that can be prepared the night before. Dietary fiber: 2 grams.

4	slices whole-wheat bread, cubed	2	cups 1% milk
4	slices Canadian bacon, chopped	1	teaspoon Worcestershire sauce
2	ounces shredded low-fat Cheddar cheese	1	teaspoon prepared mustard
4	eggs	½	teaspoon curry powder

Preheat oven to 350° F.

Coat a 9-inch-square nonstick pan with cooking spray. Spread the bread cubes over the bottom of the pan. Sprinkle with the chopped Canadian bacon and cheese.

In a medium bowl, beat the eggs, milk, Worcestershire sauce, mustard, and curry powder. Pour the egg mixture over the cheese and bread. Mixture can be covered and refrigerated overnight or baked immediately.

Bake uncovered until the eggs are set, about 30 minutes.

Per Serving: 257 Calories; 10g Fat (34.6% calories from fat); 22g Protein; 20g Carbohydrate; 209mg Cholesterol; 779mg Sodium. Exchanges: 1 Grain (Starch); 2 Lean Meat; ½ Non-Fat Milk; 1 Fat; 0 Other Carbohydrates.

Apple-Cinnamon Oatmeal

Servings: 2

Oatmeal never tasted so good! Dietary fiber: 4 grams.

1 cup unsweetened apple juice	¾ cup rolled oats
½ cup water	⅓ cup 1% milk
½ teaspoon ground cinnamon	2 tablespoons chopped walnuts
⅛ teaspoon salt	

In a small saucepan, heat apple juice, water, cinnamon, and salt until boiling. Stir in oats; lower heat and cook for five minutes, stirring occasionally.

Heat the milk. Spoon the cooked oat mixture into serving bowls. Pour on the hot milk and sprinkle with walnuts.

Per Serving: 241 Calories; 7g Fat (25.1% calories from fat); 8g Protein; 38g Carbohydrate; 2mg Cholesterol; 161mg Sodium. Exchanges: 1½ Grain (Starch); 0 Lean Meat; 1 Fruit; 0 Non-Fat Milk; 1 Fat.

Cheese and Tomato Omelet

Servings: 1

A quick breakfast, lunch, or dinner meal. Dietary fiber: 1 gram.

1	teaspoon canola oil	2	medium eggs
1	tablespoon chopped green onions	¼	teaspoon salt
¼	cup chopped tomatoes	¼	teaspoon pepper
¼	cup sliced mushrooms (optional)	1	ounce shredded cheddar cheese

Heat oil in a small nonstick skillet. Sauté onions, tomatoes, and mushrooms over medium heat until soft, about 3 minutes. Remove vegetables from skillet and set aside. Beat eggs in a small bowl; add salt and pepper. Pour the eggs into the skillet and stir until they begin to set, about 10 seconds.

Pull cooked eggs from the sides of the pan toward the center with a spatula to allow the uncooked egg to run underneath. Continue until eggs are cooked.

Spoon the vegetable filling mixture onto the center. Sprinkle the cheddar cheese on top. Flip one side of the omelet toward the center with a spatula to fold in half. Slide the omelet onto a serving plate.

Serving Idea: Spoon fresh tomato salsa on top. Serve with fresh steamed asparagus for a lunch or dinner meal.

Per Serving: 303 Calories; 23g Fat (68.3% calories from fat); 19g Protein; 5g Carbohydrate; 404mg Cholesterol; 826mg Sodium. Exchanges: 0 Grain (Starch); 2½ Lean Meat; ½ Vegetable; 3 Fat.

Whole-Wheat Buttermilk Pancakes

Servings: 6

Prepare ahead of time for a nutritious breakfast treat. Dietary fiber: 5 grams.

1½ cups rolled oats		1	cup whole-wheat flour
2 cups low-fat buttermilk		2	teaspoons baking soda
½ cup 1% milk		3	packets Splenda or other
2 eggs, beaten			non-caloric sweetener

Combine oats, buttermilk, lowfat milk, and eggs and let stand for ½ hour or overnight in refrigerator.

Add flour, baking soda, and Splenda; stir until dry ingredients are mixed well. Spray a medium nonstick skillet with cooking oil and preheat. Small amounts of additional lowfat milk can be stirred into batter if it is too thick. However, whole-wheat batter will be thicker in consistency than white flour batter and should be watched carefully while cooking to prevent burning.

Spoon ½ cup of batter onto the preheated skillet and cook over medium heat until pancake is lightly brown and firm on cooked side. Turn pancake and cook through.

Top with sugar-free maple syrup, Polaner fruit spread, or fresh fruit.

Variations: Add ¾ cup chopped nuts or ¾ cup fresh or frozen blueberries to batter when flour is added.

Per Serving: 238 Calories; 5g Fat (19.6% calories from fat); 12g Protein; 37g Carbohydrate; 66mg Cholesterol; 743mg Sodium. Exchanges: 2 Grain (Starch); ½ Lean Meat; ½ Non-Fat Milk; 1 Fat.

Soups

Southwestern-Style Black Bean Soup

Servings: 6

Try doubling the recipe of this flavorful soup—leftovers taste great, since time improves the flavor. Dietary fiber: 9 grams.

1½ cups dried black beans, soaked and drained	1 jalapeño pepper, seeded and chopped
6 cups water	2 teaspoons ground cumin
2 tablespoons olive oil	1 teaspoon ground coriander
1 large onion, chopped	2 teaspoons dried oregano
1 red bell pepper, seeded and chopped	1 teaspoon dried thyme
½ cup chopped celery	½ teaspoon ground black pepper
4 garlic cloves, minced	½ cup canned diced tomatoes
	2 teaspoons salt
	4 chopped green onions

Soak beans according to package directions.

Place the drained, soaked beans in a medium saucepan, add water, and cook for 45 minutes. Drain, reserving 4 cups of the cooking liquid. Set aside.

Heat the oil in a medium saucepan and add the onion, bell pepper, celery, garlic, and jalapeño. Sauté for 8 minutes over medium heat, or until the vegetables are tender.

Add the beans, cooking liquid, cumin, coriander, oregano, thyme, and black pepper. Cook, simmering for about 20 minutes, stirring occasionally.

Stir in the diced tomatoes and salt. Cook for an additional 15 minutes. For a thicker soup, purée half of the soup in a blender, or mash some of the beans through a sieve, and return to the pan.

Sprinkle green onions over the top for a garnish.

Serving Idea: Top each serving with a teaspoon of light sour cream.

Per Serving: 234 Calories; 6g Fat (20.6% calories from fat); 12g Protein; 37g Carbohydrate; 0mg Cholesterol; 734mg Sodium. Exchanges: 2 Grain (Starch); ½ Lean Meat; 1 Vegetable; 1 Fat.

Chicken Sausage Gumbo

Servings: 8

This gumbo takes time to prepare, but it is well worth the effort—make it a family weekend endeavor. Dietary fiber: 6 grams.

2½	pounds skinless chicken breasts (bone-in)	1	15-ounce can diced tomatoes, undrained
12	cups water	½	pound light smoked or andouille sausage
2	tablespoons canola oil	1	bay leaf
1½	pounds okra, sliced thin	1	teaspoon dried basil
¼	cup canola oil	1	teaspoon dried thyme
¼	cup whole-wheat flour	1	teaspoon cayenne pepper
1	large onion, chopped	1	teaspoon black pepper
1	medium green bell pepper, chopped	1	teaspoon salt
2	celery ribs, chopped	4	cups cooked brown rice
4	garlic cloves, chopped		

Poach chicken in water until tender and easily removed from bones, about 1 hour, skimming fat and foam from the surface of the water.

Reserve stock and allow chicken to cool. Remove the meat from the bones and set meat aside, discarding the bones.

Meanwhile, sauté the okra in 2 tablespoons of oil for about 15 minutes or enough time to eliminate ropiness.

In large Dutch oven, heat ¼ cup oil. Slowly add the flour and cook over medium heat, stirring constantly to make a brown roux, about 15 to 20 minutes. Add onion, bell pepper, celery, and garlic and sauté until vegetables are tender, about 15 minutes. Add okra, tomatoes, sausage, bay leaf, basil, thyme, cayenne, black pepper, and salt.

Add the reserved chicken stock; mix well and bring to a boil. Simmer for 1 hour with the pot loosely covered, stirring occasionally.

Add cooked chicken and simmer for an additional 15 minutes. Serve over basmati or brown rice.

Per Serving: 450 Calories; 17g Fat (33.4% calories from fat); 36g Protein; 39g Carbohydrate; 83mg Cholesterol; 713mg Sodium. Exchanges: 1½ Grain (Starch); 3½ Lean Meat; 2 Vegetable; 2 Fat.

Italian Lentil Soup

Servings: 4

This tasty soup boasts a lot of flavor and nutrition with a short preparation and cooking time. Dietary fiber: 9 grams.

½ cup dried lentils,
    rinsed and picked clean
8 cups water, divided
12 ounces spinach leaves,
    rinsed and drained
1 teaspoon olive oil
½ pound Italian sausage,
    casing removed, sliced
    into ¼-inch-thick pieces

1 medium onion, chopped
3 teaspoons low-sodium
    chicken bouillon granules
⅛ teaspoon hot pepper flakes
4 tablespoons Parmesan cheese,
    grated

Combine lentils and 4 cups water in a saucepan; simmer uncovered 20 minutes or until tender. Drain.

Cut off spinach stems and discard. Chop leaves coarsely.

Heat oil in a 4-quart pot over medium heat. Add sausage and cook, breaking it into small pieces with a wooden spoon. Cook sausage 3 minutes or until no longer pink, stirring constantly. Add onion and spinach and cook 3 minutes or until spinach is wilted. Add the chicken bouillon granules and 4 cups of water. Bring to a boil; lower heat and simmer, covered, for 15 minutes.

Add lentils and red pepper flakes. Simmer 3 minutes more.

Ladle into 4 bowls. Top with Parmesan cheese.

Per Serving: 334 Calories; 21g Fat (55.5% calories from fat); 19g Protein; 19g Carbohydrate; 47mg Cholesterol; 574mg Sodium. Exchanges: 1 Grain (Starch); 2 Lean Meat; 1 Vegetable; 3 Fat.

Artichoke Soup

Servings: 6

A delicious blend of flavors that will become a favorite of both family and guests. Dietary fiber: 8 grams.

¼ cup olive oil

2 tablespoons margarine

1 medium onion, chopped

5 garlic cloves, minced

2 14-ounce cans artichoke
   hearts, drained and quartered

1 tablespoon chopped fresh parsley

2 teaspoons dried oregano

¼ teaspoon Tabasco sauce

1 teaspoon lemon juice

½ teaspoon salt

1 10½-ounce can cream of
   chicken soup

2 tablespoons whole-wheat flour

4 low-sodium chicken
   bouillon cubes

4 cups water, divided

In a large saucepan, sauté onion and garlic in oil and margarine until soft. Add artichoke hearts; cook until soft. Add parsley, oregano, Tabasco sauce, lemon juice, and salt.

Add cream of chicken soup with one cup of water. Stir until well blended.

Heat three cups of water and blend in the whole-wheat flour until well mixed; add the chicken bouillon cubes, mashing with a fork. Combine flour mixture with artichoke mixture in saucepan and stir. Bring to boil; lower heat, cover, and cook on low heat for 1 hour, stirring occasionally.

Per Serving: 216 Calories; 15g Fat (56.4% calories from fat); 6g Protein; 19g Carbohydrate; 2mg Cholesterol; 554mg Sodium. Exchanges: ½ Grain (Starch); 3 Vegetable; 0 Fruit; 3 Fat.

Broccoli Pasta Soup

Servings: 6

This great tasting soup can be prepared and cooked in minutes. Dietary fiber: 4 grams.

3   10½-ounce cans chicken broth
4   garlic cloves, minced
2   teaspoons dried thyme
3   cups broccoli florets,
        broken into 1-inch pieces

6   ounces uncooked whole-wheat
        fusilli pasta
3   teaspoons grated Parmesan
        cheese (optional)

SOUPS

In medium pan, heat chicken broth, garlic, and thyme until boiling. Add broccoli and fusilli. Reduce heat and cook until broccoli is tender and pasta is cooked al dente, about 10 minutes.

Spoon soup into individual serving bowls and sprinkle each with ½ teaspoon Parmesan cheese.

Variation: Use canned vegetable broth instead of chicken broth for a vegetarian dish.

Per Serving: 141 Calories; 2g Fat (9.9% calories from fat); 9g Protein; 25g Carbohydrate; 1mg Cholesterol; 502mg Sodium. Exchanges: 1½ Grain (Starch); ½ Lean Meat; ½ Vegetable; 0 Fat.

Salads

Green Salad with Tomatoes, Cucumbers, and Creole Mustard Dressing

Servings: 4

Colorful and tangy. Dietary fiber: 2 grams.

4	cups any type lettuce leaves	1	tablespoon red wine vinegar
1	tomato, diced	1	tablespoon balsamic vinegar
1	cucumber, peeled and sliced	2	tablespoons Creole mustard
4	tablespoons olive oil		

Mix lettuce, tomato, and cucumber in large salad bowl. Chill until ready to serve.

Combine olive oil, vinegars, and Creole mustard; stir to mix well.

Pour dressing over salad just before serving, tossing to coat vegetables.

Per Serving: 143 Calories; 14g Fat (83.0% calories from fat); 1g Protein; 5g Carbohydrate; 0mg Cholesterol; 9mg Sodium. Exchanges: 1 Vegetable; 0 Fruit; 2½ Fat; 0 Other Carbohydrates.

Mediterranean Spinach Salad

Servings: 4

Dietary fiber: 2 grams.

4 cups spinach leaves	4 tablespoons olive oil
½ cup sliced black olives	4 tablespoons red wine vinegar
2 ounces crumbled feta cheese	¼ teaspoon salt
1 cup diced tomatoes	¼ teaspoon freshly ground black pepper

Wash and dry spinach leaves. Remove the stems and discard them; chop spinach into bite-sized pieces.

Add black olives, feta cheese, and tomatoes and mix.

Combine olive oil, vinegar, salt, and pepper; mix well.

Pour dressing over spinach mixture just before serving.

Per Serving: 195 Calories; 19g Fat (82.1% calories from fat); 3g Protein; 6g Carbohydrate; 13mg Cholesterol; 467mg Sodium. Exchanges: 0 Grain (Starch); ½ Lean Meat; ½ Vegetable; 0 Fruit; 3½ Fat; 0 Other Carbohydrates.

SALADS

Light Caesar Salad with Grilled Chicken Strips

Servings: 6

This light version of the classic is low in fat but just as delicious. Dietary fiber: 2 grams.

3	tablespoons lemon juice	1	teaspoon salt
1	teaspoon lemon zest	1	recipe Grilled Chicken
3	garlic cloves, minced		(see p. 147)
2	teaspoons white wine vinegar	1	large head romaine lettuce,
4	ounces extra-virgin olive oil		rinsed, patted dry, torn into
1	teaspoon freshly ground		pieces, and chilled
	black pepper	2	ounces grated Parmesan cheese

(see p. 147)

Combine the lemon juice and lemon zest, garlic, and vinegar in a small bowl, and mix well. Add the olive oil, whisking well until mixture is smooth. Add the pepper and salt and set aside.

When ready to serve, slice the Grilled Chicken into ¼-inch-wide strips. Combine lettuce with Caesar dressing, mixing well to coat leaves. Add Grilled Chicken strips, stirring well.

Serve on individual plates topped with freshly grated Parmesan cheese.

Per Serving: 419 Calories; 26g Fat (56.1% calories from fat); 41g Protein; 5g Carbohydrate; 103mg Cholesterol; 626mg Sodium. Exchanges: 5½ Lean Meat; 1 Vegetable; 0 Fruit; 4 Fat.

SALADS

Mandarin Orange Salad

Servings: 6

This refreshing salad is light and easy to prepare and is a Sugar Busters version of the Del Monte recipe that appears on their canned mandarins. Dietary fiber: 2 grams.

6   cups torn lettuce leaves
1   15-ounce can mandarin oranges
    in water, drained (If mandarin
    oranges packed in water are not
    available, drain and rinse
    mandarin oranges packed
    in light syrup.)

½   medium red onion, sliced
⅓   cup olive oil
¼   cup white wine vinegar
1   tablespoon Dijon mustard
⅓   cup halved and toasted walnuts

Combine lettuce, oranges, and onion in salad bowl.

Blend together oil, vinegar, and mustard.

Add nuts and toss dressing with salad just before serving.

Per Serving: 197 Calories; 16g Fat (70.9% calories from fat); 3g Protein; 12g Carbohydrate; 0mg Cholesterol; 43mg Sodium. Exchanges: 0 Grain (Starch); 0 Lean Meat; ½ Vegetable; ½ Fruit; 3 Fat; 0 Other Carbohydrates.

SALADS

Curried Tuna Salad

Servings: 4

A slight change of pace from the usual tuna salad. Dietary fiber: trace.

1 12-ounce can tuna	½ teaspoon curry powder
packed in water, drained	¼ teaspoon salt
⅓ cup finely chopped celery	⅛ teaspoon ground ginger
4 ounces plain nonfat yogurt	Dash red pepper

Combine all ingredients. Mix well and chill.

Serving Ideas: Serve over lettuce leaves or in a whole-wheat bread sandwich topped with lettuce.

Per Serving: 117 Calories; 1g Fat (6.4% calories from fat); 23g Protein; 3g Carbohydrate; 26mg Cholesterol; 451mg Sodium. Exchanges: 0 Grain (Starch); 3 Lean Meat; 0 Vegetable; 0 Non-Fat Milk; 0 Fat.

SALADS

Tabbouleh

Servings: 6

A refreshing traditional Lebanese salad. Dietary fiber: 5 grams.

1   cup bulgur
1   cup hot water
½   cup finely chopped parsley
½   cup finely chopped red onion
½   cup finely chopped fresh
      mint leaves
2   garlic cloves, finely minced
¼   cup fresh lemon juice
⅓   cup extra-virgin olive oil
1   teaspoon salt
½   teaspoon freshly ground
      black pepper
1   large ripe tomato,
      seeded and diced

Put the bulgur in a large bowl, cover with hot water, and soak at room temperature for 40 minutes to 1 hour until most of the water is absorbed and the bulgur is tender. Pour off any remaining water. Fluff with a fork.

Stir in the parsley, red onion, mint, and garlic. Toss with a fork.

Add the lemon juice, olive oil, salt, and pepper and mix.

Add the tomato and toss again. Let stand for 20 minutes.

Serving Idea: Serve on a platter surrounded by crisp romaine lettuce leaves to use as scoops.

Per Serving: 205 Calories; 12g Fat (52.1% calories from fat); 4g Protein; 22g Carbohydrate; 0mg Cholesterol; 368mg Sodium. Exchanges: 1 Grain (Starch); ½ Vegetable; 0 Fruit; 2½ Fat.

French Dressing

Yield: 1 cup dressing

Serve over green salad or fresh fruit. Dietary fiber: 2 grams.

½ teaspoon unflavored gelatin
1 tablespoon cold water
¼ cup boiling water
½ cup tomato juice
3 tablespoons vinegar
1 teaspoon Splenda or other
    non-caloric sweetener (optional)

1 tablespoon Worcestershire sauce
½ teaspoon salt
¼ teaspoon dry mustard
⅛ teaspoon garlic powder
¼ teaspoon pepper

SALADS

Dissolve gelatin in cold water. Add boiling water; stir gelatin well and set aside.

Combine remaining ingredients in container of electric blender or food processor; process for about 20 seconds. Add gelatin mixture; process until smooth. Chill thoroughly. Stir well before serving.

Per Serving: 9 Calories; trace Fat (2.9% calories from fat); trace Protein; 2g Carbohydrate; 0mg Cholesterol; 277mg Sodium. Exchanges: 0 Grain (Starch); 0 Lean Meat; 0 Vegetable; 0 Fat; 0 Other Carbohydrates.

Balsalmic Vinegar Dressing

Yield: ⅔ cup

6	tablespoons balsamic vinegar	2	garlic cloves, minced
4	tablespoons olive oil	½	teaspoon dried thyme
4	tablespoons lemon juice		

Combine ingredients and mix well. Chill for at least 20 minutes.

Per Serving: 129 Calories; 14g Fat (89.5% calories from fat); trace Protein; 3g Carbohydrate; 0mg Cholesterol; 1mg Sodium. Exchanges: 0 Grain (Starch); 0 Vegetable; 0 Fruit; 2½ Fat.

SALADS

Tofu Garlic Dressing

Yield: ¾ cup

A creamy dressing that provides an easy way to add soy to your diet. Dietary fiber: trace.

6   ounces silken tofu (Mori-Nu
    brand is recommended)
2   tablespoons tarragon vinegar
2   tablespoons extra-virgin olive oil

1   garlic clove, minced
2   tablespoons grated
    Parmesan cheese
¼   teaspoon salt

Combine tofu, vinegar, olive oil, garlic, cheese, and salt in a food processor or blender and blend until smooth.

Variation: Omit Parmesan cheese and add ½ teaspoon of dried or fresh herbs of your choice.

Serving Idea: Serve over sliced tomatoes, mushrooms, and greens.

Per Serving: 70 Calories; 6g Fat (77.9% calories from fat); 3g Protein; 1g Carbohydrate; 1mg Cholesterol; 122mg Sodium. Exchanges: ½ Lean Meat; 0 Vegetable; 1 Fat; 0 Other Carbohydrates.

Main Dishes

Terrific Turkey Burgers

Servings: 4

These well-seasoned burgers are kid pleasers. Dietary fiber: 3 grams.

1 tablespoon canola oil	8 ounces canned kidney beans, rinsed and drained
1 medium onion, finely chopped	
2 cloves garlic, finely chopped	4 tablespoons sugar-free ketchup
1 teaspoon chili powder	1 teaspoon salt
1 teaspoon ground cumin	½ teaspoon pepper
1 pound ground turkey	

In a medium frying pan, heat the canola oil and cook the onion for 5 minutes, until it begins to brown. Add the garlic, chili powder, and cumin and sauté for 2 minutes. Remove from the heat and let cool completely.

Place the ground turkey, kidney beans, and ketchup in a large bowl. Stir in the cooled onion mixture and mix well. Shape the turkey mixture into four patties.

Cook on outdoor grill or broil in a preheated oven, cooking for about 15 minutes, or until the burgers are cooked thoroughly, turning halfway through the cooking time.

Serving Idea: Serve with lettuce, sliced tomatoes, and sugar-free plain yogurt or mustard on a whole-wheat bun.

Per Serving: 262 Calories; 13g Fat (45.7% calories from fat); 23g Protein; 12g Carbohydrate; 90mg Cholesterol; 845mg Sodium. Exchanges: ½ Grain (Starch); 3 Lean Meat; ½ Vegetable; 1 Fat.

MAIN DISHES

Crock-Pot Beef Roast

Servings: 8

An easy and tender roast dish that can be cooked longer and shredded for serving as sloppy joes on wheat buns. Dietary fiber: 2 grams.

1	3-pound eye round roast	1	large onion, sliced
1	teaspoon salt	1	10½-ounce can onion soup
1	teaspoon freshly ground	1	10½-ounce can cream
	black pepper		of mushroom soup
1	tablespoon olive oil	3	cups cooked brown rice

Season the roast with salt and pepper. Heat the olive oil in a large skillet and lightly brown the roast on all sides. Place the roast in Crock-Pot. (The roast can be cut in half for quicker cooking.)

Add the sliced onion to the skillet and sauté in oil for about 3 minutes. Add the onion and mushroom soup. Stir well. Bring to simmer and pour mixture over roast in Crock-Pot. Add enough water just to cover roast. Cook for 3 to 4 hours until roast is tender. Or cook 5 to 6 hours so that roast can be shredded for sloppy joes.

Variations: If you do not have a Crock-Pot, roast beef in 350° F oven, covered, for 2 to 2½ hours or until fork-tender.

Serving Ideas: Slice roast and spoon the sauce over cooked brown rice. Serve with steamed green beans.

Per Serving: 368 Calories; 22g Fat (53.8% calories from fat); 21g Protein; 19g Carbohydrate; 66 mg Cholesterol; 622mg Sodium. Exchanges: 1 Grain (Starch); 2½ Lean Meat; 1½ Vegetable; 2½ Fat.

MAIN DISHES

Taco Salad

Servings: 6

For a great Sugar Busters meal, forget the traditional corn chips and spoon beef sauce over crisp lettuce. Dietary fiber: 2 grams.

1½ pounds extra-lean ground beef
1 medium onion, chopped
4 cloves garlic, chopped
¼ teaspoon cayenne pepper
½ teaspoon salt
¼ teaspoon black pepper
½ teaspoon ground cumin

1 teaspoon chili powder
1 15-ounce can tomato sauce
4 cups romaine lettuce, cut into
   ½-inch strips across the width
6 tablespoons grated low-fat
   Cheddar cheese
2 cups Tomato Salsa
   (see page 187)

Spray a medium nonstick or iron skillet with nonstick vegetable cooking spray, and heat. Add ground beef, onion, and garlic. Cook over medium heat until meat is browned and cooked thoroughly, about 10 minutes.

Drain oil from meat mixture and return meat to heat. Add cayenne pepper, salt, black pepper, cumin, chili powder, and tomato sauce. Mix well and simmer over low heat for 20 to 30 minutes, stirring frequently.

Arrange lettuce on individual dinner plates. Spoon on meat sauce. Top with Tomato Salsa (page 187) or bottled salsa. Sprinkle each serving with 1 tablespoon cheese.

Per Serving: 316 Calories; 20g Fat (57.7% calories from fat); 24g Protein; 9g Carbohydrate; 79mg Cholesterol; 713mg Sodium. Exchanges: 0 Grain (Starch); 3 Lean Meat; 1½ Vegetable; 2 Fat.

MAIN DISHES

Italian Meat Roll

Servings: 8

This spicy meat loaf should please the family. Dietary fiber: 2 grams.

1   cup whole-wheat breadcrumbs
2   eggs, beaten
2   tablespoons chopped fresh parsley
½ cup no-salt tomato juice
½ teaspoon salt
½ teaspoon black pepper

2   cloves garlic, minced
½ teaspoon dried oregano
2   pounds lean ground beef
6   lean ham slices
6   ounces shredded mozzarella
    cheese

Preheat oven to 350° F.

Combine breadcrumbs, eggs, parsley, tomato juice, salt, black pepper, garlic, and oregano in a medium bowl and stir. Add ground beef and mix well.

On sheet of wax paper or foil, flatten meat mixture into a 12 × 10–inch rectangle.

Layer ham slices on top of meat and top with shredded cheese, leaving a small border of meat on the edge.

Roll up meat, starting from the short edge and lifting the wax paper to aid in rolling; press roll together at edges.

Place seam-side down on a baking sheet and bake for 60 to 75 minutes until done.

Cut meat loaf into 1-inch medallions.

Note: If whole-wheat breadcrumbs are unavailable, place 4 slices of day-old wheat bread in a food processor and process on high.

Per Serving: 468 Calories; 32g Fat (61.9% calories from fat); 32g Protein; 12g Carbohydrate; 161mg Cholesterol; 597mg Sodium. Exchanges: ½ Grain (Starch); 4½ Lean Meat; 0 Vegetable; 4 Fat.

Tofu Chili Tortillas

Servings: 6

A meatless meal that combines the kid-pleasing taste of chili with the health benefits of vegetables and tofu. Dietary fiber: 5 grams.

2 tablespoons olive oil	¼ teaspoon ground cumin
2 cups broccoli florets, cut into ½-inch pieces	¼ teaspoon ground black pepper
	2 teaspoons chili powder
1 cup sliced mushrooms	12 ounces firm or extra-firm tofu,
1 medium yellow onion, chopped	cut into ½-inch cubes
4 garlic cloves, minced	6 whole-wheat tortillas
15 ounces tomato sauce	2 ounces shredded low-fat
¼ teaspoon Tabasco sauce	Cheddar cheese

Preheat oven to 350° F.

In a large nonstick skillet, heat oil over medium heat. Add the broccoli, mushrooms, onion, and garlic. Cook over medium-high heat, stirring frequently, until vegetables are tender, about 8 minutes.

Meanwhile, in a small bowl, combine the tomato sauce, Tabasco, cumin, pepper, and chili powder; add the mixture to the skillet and stir to coat vegetables.

Stir the tofu into the skillet gently to prevent the cubes from breaking. Cover and heat 5 minutes over medium-low heat.

Place the tortillas on a cookie sheet that has been lightly sprayed with nonstick cooking spray; toast until crispy, about 3 minutes on each side.

Spoon tofu chili onto center of each tortilla; sprinkle with cheese, roll up, and serve.

Variations: A 15-ounce can of rinsed and drained black beans can be added to the recipe to boost the fiber content, or you can serve this nutritious chili over hot basmati or brown rice.

Per Serving: 378 Calories; 13g Fat (30.7% calories from fat); 15g Protein; 52g Carbohydrate; 2mg Cholesterol; 853mg Sodium. Exchanges: 3 Grain (Starch); 1½ Lean Meat; 1½ Vegetable; 2 Fat.

MAIN DISHES

Quesadillas

Servings: 4

Something different for lunch. Dietary fiber: 3 grams.

4   6-inch whole-wheat tortillas
4   ounces lowfat shredded
    Cheddar cheese
4   ounces shredded Monterey
    Jack cheese

1   cup diced tomatoes
4   tablespoons chopped green
    onions
4   tablespoons sour cream
4   ounces Tomato Salsa
    (see page 187)

Place an individual tortilla in a warm nonstick skillet.

Cover with ¼ of the cheese, tomatoes, and onions. Cook on one side until cheese is melted.

Cut into 4 wedges and garnish with sour cream and salsa.

Per Serving: 440 Calories; 19g Fat (39.8% calories from fat); 21g Protein; 44g Carbohydrate; 38mg Cholesterol; 684mg Sodium. Exchanges: 2½ Grain (Starch); 2 Lean Meat; ½ Vegetable; 0 Nonfat Milk; 2½ Fat.

Grilled Chicken

Servings: 4

Easily prepared and with a large variety of seasoning choices, grilled chicken is a versatile choice as the basis for numerous dishes. Dietary fiber: 1 gram.

4	skinless, boneless chicken breasts	4	cloves garlic, minced
½	teaspoon salt	2	rosemary sprigs, leaves removed
¼	teaspoon black pepper		and chopped or 1 teaspoon
3	tablespoons low-calorie		dried
	Italian salad dressing		

Salt and pepper chicken breasts. Place in shallow baking dish. Pour on salad dressing. Turn to coat all sides.

Sprinkle garlic and rosemary on chicken, rubbing on spices to cover all sides evenly. Marinate in refrigerator for 30 minutes or more.

Remove chicken from marinade and drain. Discard marinade. Place chicken on hot grill and grill until chicken is cooked through but still moist, about 2 to 5 minutes on each side, depending on thickness.

Variations: Chicken can be grilled indoors in a grilling machine that cooks foods on both sides at once. This helpful and popular small appliance allows fat to drain off, and cooks ground meat patties, chicken, and fish filets in a very short time with good results. You can also broil marinated chicken in oven, turning once.

Serving Ideas: Grilled chicken filets can be cut into strips and served as fajitas, added to salads to convert them to entrées, or combined with pasta and rice dishes.

Per Serving: 301 Calories; 7g Fat (23.3% calories from fat); 53g Protein; 3g Carbohydrate; 145mg Cholesterol; 481mg Sodium. Exchanges: 0 Grain (Starch); 7½ Lean Meat; 0 Vegetable; ½ Fat; 0 Other Carbohydrates.

MAIN DISHES

Oven-Fried Chicken

Servings: 4

You don't need oil or flour to prepare crispy, crunchy chicken. Dietary fiber: 2 grams.

2   pounds skinless, boneless
      chicken breasts
2   teaspoons Creole seasoning
2   cups Wheaties
½   teaspoon garlic powder

2   tablespoons sesame seeds
      (optional)
1   tablespoon Worcestershire sauce
¾   cup low-fat buttermilk

Preheat the oven to 350° F.

Wash chicken breasts and pat dry. Season chicken with Creole seasoning or if you prefer, salt and pepper. Set aside.

Pour Wheaties into a large plastic Ziploc bag. Close, removing air from the bag. Crush the Wheaties with a rolling pin, being careful not to make the coating too fine. Add the garlic powder and sesame seeds to the Wheaties and shake the bag to mix well.

In a shallow bowl, combine the buttermilk and Worcestershire sauce; mix and set aside.

Spray a large baking sheet with nonstick cooking spray. Set aside.

Pour the Wheaties mixture onto a large plate. Dip the chicken pieces first in the buttermilk; coat well on all sides. Then dredge the chicken in the Wheaties mixture.

Arrange the chicken pieces on the coated baking sheet. Spray the chicken lightly with nonstick cooking spray. Bake for 30 minutes or until golden brown.

Variations: Skinless bone-in chicken pieces can be substituted for the chicken breasts, if you like. If so, the cooking time should be increased. Experiment with the family's favorite spices, perhaps dried rosemary, to coat the chicken. Or substitute low-fat milk mixed with one egg for the buttermilk as a coating.

Per Serving: 376 Calories; 9g Fat (22.2% calories from fat); 55g Protein; 17g Carbohydrate; 140mg Cholesterol; 423mg Sodium. Exchanges: 1 Grain (Starch); 7 Lean Meat; 0 Nonfat Milk; ½ Fat; 0 Other Carbohydrates.

MAIN DISHES

Grilled Chicken and Mandarin Salad

Servings: 4

A refreshing light meal, especially enjoyable as a summer lunch or dinner. Dietary fiber: 5 grams.

1	large head romaine lettuce, rinsed, patted dry, torn into pieces, and chilled	1	recipe Grilled Chicken (see page 147)
2	tablespoons olive oil	1	14-ounce can mandarin oranges in light syrup, drained and rinsed
2	tablespoons rice wine vinegar		
½	teaspoon salt	1	cup French Dressing
¼	teaspoon black pepper		(see page 138)

Slice prepared Grilled Chicken into thin strips 1/4 inch wide.

When ready to serve, toss lettuce leaves with olive oil, vinegar, salt, and pepper.

Carefully stir in mandarin orange slices; spoon lettuce onto individual plates. Top with chicken slices and French dressing.

Per Serving: 441 Calories; 13g Fat (27.1% calories from fat); 57g Protein; 25g Carbohydrate; 144mg Cholesterol; 829mg Sodium. Exchanges: 0 Grain (Starch); 7½ Lean Meat; 1 Vegetable; 1 Fruit; 1½ Fat; 0 Other Carbohydrates.

MAIN DISHES

149

Chicken Fusilli Pasta

Servings: 6

Quick to prepare and sure to please. Dietary fiber: 5 grams.

12 ounces uncooked fusilli whole-wheat pasta	½ teaspoon freshly ground black pepper
1 tablespoon butter or margarine	4 skinless, boneless chicken breasts, cut into 1-inch pieces
4 tablespoons olive oil	
2 leeks, white part only, sliced thin	½ cup chopped sun-dried tomatoes
4 cloves garlic, minced	¼ cup half-and-half
½ teaspoon red pepper flakes	3 tablespoons grated Parmesan cheese
1 teaspoon salt	

Prepare the pasta according to package directions and keep warm.

In medium skillet, melt the butter in the olive oil. Sauté the leeks with garlic, red pepper flakes, salt, and pepper. Add chicken pieces and sauté until chicken is done, about 10 minutes. Reduce the heat and add the sun-dried tomatoes and half-and-half; mix well. Cook until mixture is hot but not boiling.

Pour the warm pasta into a large serving bowl and add the chicken mixture; mix well. Top with grated Parmesan cheese.

Per serving: 526 Calories; 18g Fat (30.0% calories from fat); 45g Protein; 48g Carbohydrate; 107mg Cholesterol; 520mg Sodium. Exchanges: 3 Grain (Starch); 5 Lean Meat; 1 Vegetable; 0 Nonfat Milk; 2½ Fat.

MAIN DISHES

Chicken Fajitas

Servings: 4

Marinated and grilled chicken strips served with a variety of toppings will allow each family member to create an individualized meal. Dietary fiber: 4 grams.

4 tablespoons olive oil, divided	1½ pounds skinless, boneless
4 tablespoons lime juice	chicken breasts
1 teaspoon dried oregano	1 medium onion, halved and
½ teaspoon cumin	cut into ½-inch thick slices
2 tablespoons Worcestershire	1 bell pepper, halved and sliced
sauce	4 whole-wheat tortillas
½ teaspoon salt	2 medium tomatoes,
1 teaspoon pepper	seeded and chopped
2 garlic cloves, chopped	2 tablespoons chopped cilantro

Combine 3 tablespoons olive oil, lime juice, oregano, cumin, Worcestershire sauce, salt, pepper, and garlic. Mix well. Place chicken breasts in a shallow glass dish. Cover with marinade, coating chicken well on all sides. Cover dish and marinate in refrigerator for 1 or more hours.

After chicken has been marinated, heat the remaining 1 tablespoon olive oil in a medium nonstick skillet. Sauté onions and bell pepper in the olive oil for about 6 minutes or until tender. Remove from heat and keep warm.

Combine chopped tomatoes and cilantro. Set aside.

Remove chicken from marinade, place on a grill rack coated with vegetable spray and cook 8 minutes on each side or until chicken is done.

Heat whole-wheat tortillas wrapped in foil on the grill or wrap the tortillas in slightly moistened paper towels and microwave for 1 minute.

Cut chicken diagonally across the grain into thin slices. Place warm tortillas on a plate. Arrange chicken on a large platter and cover with the onion and bell pepper mixture. Spoon chicken mixture onto tortillas, cover with tomato salsa. Fold sides of tortilla over filling.

Serving Idea: Low-fat sour cream or ½ cup grated Monterey Jack or reduced-fat Cheddar cheese can be added to the list of toppings.

Per Serving: 604 Calories; 24g Fat (35.2% calories from fat); 46g Protein; 52g Carbohydrate; 104mg Cholesterol; 784mg Sodium. Exchanges: 2½ Grain (Starch); 5½ Lean Meat; 1½ Vegetable; 0 Fruit; 3½ Fat; 0 Other Carbohydrates.

MAIN DISHES

151

Chicken Barley Casserole

Servings: 6

Barley takes the place of rice to give this hearty meal one-fourth of the recommended daily intake of fiber. Dietary fiber: 7 grams.

1 teaspoon ground cumin	6 chicken thighs, skin removed
1 teaspoon chili powder	2 small onions, chopped
½ teaspoon ground cinnamon	1 large red bell pepper, chopped
½ teaspoon mint flakes or 2 teaspoons chopped fresh mint	1 tablespoon low-sodium soy sauce
	3½ cups chicken broth
½ teaspoon garlic powder	1 cup uncooked barley
½ teaspoon salt	1 14½-ounce can diced tomatoes,
¼ teaspoon ground red pepper	drained
2 tablespoons canola oil, divided	6 tablespoons chopped green onions

Combine the cumin, chili powder, cinnamon, mint flakes, garlic powder, salt, and red pepper in a small bowl. Divide the mixture in half and rub the chicken thighs with half of the spice mixture.

Spray a large nonstick skillet with cooking spray and heat 1 tablespoon of the oil over medium heat. Add the chicken and cook on each side until the chicken is browned, about 2 minutes. Remove the chicken from the skillet.

Heat the remaining tablespoon of oil in the skillet. Add the onions, red pepper, and soy sauce. Cook over medium-high heat until vegetables are lightly browned, about 5 minutes.

Add the chicken broth, barley, tomatoes, and the remaining spice mixture. Mix well.

Add the chicken to the vegetable mixture. Bring to a boil, cover, reduce heat, and simmer 1 hour or until chicken is done and most of the liquid is absorbed. Sprinkle with green onions.

Per Serving: 293 Calories; 9g Fat (27.5% calories from fat); 22g Protein; 32g Carbohydrate; 57mg Cholesterol; 895mg Sodium. Exchanges: 1½ Grain (Starch); 2 Lean Meat; 1½ Vegetable; 1 Fat.

Mango Chicken

Servings: 4

This unusual combination provides light yet tasty dinner fare. Dietary fiber: 2 grams.

1 cup uncooked basmati rice, rinsed well and drained	½ teaspoon freshly ground black pepper
1½ cups chicken broth	1 cup chopped red onion
1½ pounds skinless, boneless chicken breasts	1 mango, peeled and diced into ½-inch pieces
3 tablespoons olive oil	3 tablespoons fresh lime juice
½ teaspoon salt	⅓ cup chopped cilantro

Add rinsed basmati rice to chicken broth and bring to a boil. When broth reduces to level of the rice, lower heat to a simmer, cover, and cook until liquid is absorbed and rice is tender. Remove rice from heat, fluff with a fork, and keep warm.

Season chicken with salt and pepper and 1 tablespoon olive oil or, for more flavor, follow procedure for Grilled Chicken on page 147. Cook chicken breasts in skillet over moderate heat until done, 4 to 5 minutes per side. Remove chicken from skillet. When chicken is cool enough to handle, cut into ½-inch chunks.

Add remaining 2 tablespoons olive oil to skillet in which chicken was cooked. Heat oil and sauté onion until soft, about 5 minutes.

Add the cooked rice and diced chicken to the sautéed onions. Mix well and warm over low heat.

Combine the cilantro and lime juice with the diced mango and mix well.

Remove the heated chicken and rice to a large serving dish. Add the mango mixture and serve immediately.

Per Serving: 518 Calories; 16g Fat (28.6% calories from fat); 45g Protein; 47g Carbohydrate; 104mg Cholesterol; 681mg Sodium. Exchanges: 2 Grain (Starch); 5½ Lean Meat; ½ Vegetable; ½ Fruit; 2 Fat.

MAIN DISHES

Mexican Chicken and Beans

Servings: 6

A quick-cooking and flavorful way to include beans in your diet. Dietary fiber: 8 grams.

1 tablespoon canola oil	1 15-ounce can chickpeas, rinsed and drained
1 pound boneless, skinless chicken breasts, cubed	1 teaspoon cumin
1 red onion, chopped	1 teaspoon chili powder
2 garlic cloves, chopped	½ teaspoon thyme
1 cup spicy vegetable juice	1 cup chopped green onions
1 15-ounce can black beans, rinsed and drained	1 cup shredded reduced-fat Monterey Jack cheese

Heat the oil in a large skillet. Add the chicken and cook, turning, until brown on all sides, about 6 to 8 minutes. Place chicken in a bowl and set aside.

Cook the onions and garlic in the skillet, stirring frequently, until tender, 3 to 4 minutes. Stir in the juice, beans, chickpeas, cumin, chili powder, and thyme; bring to a boil. Reduce the heat to low and simmer until the mixture thickens. Stir in the chicken; cook for 5 minutes.

Sprinkle with onions and cheese before serving.

Variations: Replace the Monterey Jack cheese with low-fat cheddar. Add onions with other ingredients before the 15-minute cooking time for a milder flavor.

Per Serving: 328 Calories; 8g Fat (22.0% calories from fat); 30g Protein; 32g Carbohydrate; 53mg Cholesterol; 272mg Sodium. Exchanges: 1½ Grain (Starch); 3½ Lean Meat; 1 Vegetable; ½ Fat.

Chicken Cacciatore

Servings: 6

This is a light and flavorful dish that will become a family favorite. Dietary fiber: 8 grams.

6	skinless chicken breasts (bone-in)	1	32-ounce can diced tomatoes, undrained
½	teaspoon salt	1	8-ounce can tomato sauce
½	teaspoon pepper	1	4-ounce can sliced mushrooms
2	tablespoons olive oil	2	bay leaves
½	cup chopped onion	1	tablespoon Worcestershire sauce
3	garlic cloves, minced	2	teaspoons dried oregano
¼	cup chopped green pepper	12	ounces uncooked whole-wheat angel hair pasta
¼	cup chopped celery		

Wash chicken breasts and pat dry. Season with salt and pepper.

Heat olive oil in large Dutch oven and sauté chicken pieces until lightly browned. Remove chicken pieces and set aside.

In remaining oil, sauté the onion, garlic, green pepper, and celery for about 3 minutes, scraping bottom of pan to loosen any chicken pieces.

Add the diced tomatoes, tomato sauce, mushrooms, bay leaves, Worcestershire sauce, and oregano. Bring to a boil. Add chicken; cover, reduce heat, and simmer 30 minutes. Uncover and simmer an additional 20 to 30 minutes until chicken is tender. Discard bay leaves.

Remove cooked chicken breasts; let cool and then remove meat from bones, tearing chicken into two-inch pieces. Return deboned chicken to sauce in pan. During last 10 minutes of cooking chicken prepare angel hair pasta according to package instructions. Drain and keep warm. Spoon chicken and tomato sauce over hot angel hair pasta.

Variation: To save time, purchase boneless chicken breasts; season but do not sauté in olive oil. Omit olive oil. Combine all ingredients but chicken and pasta. Bring to boil; add chicken. Simmer covered 15 minutes and uncovered another 15 to 20 minutes or until chicken is cooked thoroughly.

Per Serving: 478 Calories; 10g Fat (17.6% calories from fat); 46g Protein; 56g Carbohydrate; 94mg Cholesterol; 827mg Sodium. Exchanges: 3 Grain (Starch); 5 Lean Meat; 2 Vegetable; 1 Fat; 0 Other Carbohydrates.

MAIN DISHES

Chicken Portobello

Servings: 6

This blend of flavors will impress family and guests. Longer cooking increases this recipe's flavor. Dietary fiber: 3 grams.

4	skinless chicken breasts	8	garlic cloves, chopped
4	skinless chicken thighs	3	leeks, white part only, thinly sliced
½	teaspoon salt		
½	teaspoon pepper	3	portobello mushrooms, chopped into large chunks
1	teaspoon Creole seasoning		
4	tablespoons olive oil	1	cup chicken broth
4	sprigs rosemary, chopped	2	tablespoons low-sodium soy sauce

Preheat oven to 350° F.

    Wash chicken pieces and pat dry with paper towels. Season chicken with salt, pepper, and Creole seasoning.

    Heat olive oil in medium skillet and lightly brown chicken on all sides, adding small amounts of additional olive oil if needed. Remove chicken from skillet and place in a shallow baking pan that has been lightly sprayed with cooking spray. Add rosemary, garlic, leeks, and mushrooms to skillet and sauté in the olive oil and remaining pan juices for two to three minutes, stirring constantly. Add chicken broth and soy sauce, stirring and scraping pan to deglaze.

    Pour portobello sauce evenly over chicken. Bake covered for 60 to 90 minutes. Place cooked chicken on serving dish and spoon sauce evenly over chicken.

Serving Ideas: Serve with steamed green vegetables or a salad.

Variations: Add two medium, peeled sweet potatoes, sliced into one-inch chunks, before baking for a meal in one dish.

Per Serving: 379 Calories; 14g Fat (33.0% calories from fat); 49g Protein; 14g Carbohydrate; 129mg Cholesterol; 696mg Sodium. Exchanges: 0 Grain (Starch); 6½ Lean Meat; 2½ Vegetable; 2 Fat; 0 Other Carbohydrates.

MAIN DISHES

Basic Tomato Sauce

Servings: 6

Use this quick sauce on whole-wheat pasta or pizza dough. Baking soda replaces the sugar traditionally used to lessen the acidic taste of the tomatoes. Dietary fiber: 2 grams.

1	medium onion, chopped	1	15-ounce can no-sugar-added
3	cloves garlic, minced		tomato sauce
3	tablespoons extra-virgin olive oil,	2	teaspoons Italian seasoning
1	28-ounce can no-sugar-added	½	teaspoon baking soda
	crushed or puréed tomatoes		Salt and pepper, to taste

In a medium skillet, sauté the onion and garlic in the olive oil until tender, about 6 minutes.

Over medium heat, add the crushed tomatoes and tomato sauce, stirring to mix.

Add the Italian seasoning and baking soda while continuing to stir.

Lower heat to a simmer.

Add salt and pepper to taste.

Simmer for 20 to 30 minutes, stirring frequently.

Per Serving: 116 Calories; 7g Fat (51.9% calories from fat); 2g Protein; 13g Carbohydrate; 0mg Cholesterol; 545mg Sodium. Exchanges: 0 Grain (Starch); 2½ Vegetable; 1½ Fat.

MAIN DISHES

Meat Sauce and Pasta

Servings: 6

A quick sauce for any shape of wheat pasta. Dietary fiber: 8 grams.

1   tablespoon olive oil
1   pound lean ground beef
1   medium onion, chopped

1   recipe Basic Tomato
    Sauce (see p 157)
12 ounces whole-wheat
    angel hair pasta

Heat oil in large, heavy skillet. Add ground beef and onion; sauté until meat is brown and cooked thoroughly. Drain excess oil.

Add one recipe of Basic Tomato Sauce that has been prepared up to the "simmer for 30 minutes" stage. Cook the combined meat and tomato sauce over medium-low heat for 30 minutes.

Prepare the pasta according to package directions. Drain.

Spoon pasta into individual serving dishes and top with meat sauce.

Variation: Add one can of red kidney beans and 2 tablespoons of chili powder during the last 20 minutes of cooking for a tasty chili that can be served over brown or basmati rice.

Per Serving: 575 Calories; 30g Fat (46.0% calories from fat); 23g Protein; 57g Carbohydrate; 64mg Cholesterol; 602mg Sodium. Exchanges: 3 Grain (Starch); 2 Lean Meat; 2½ Vegetable; 5 Fat.

MAIN DISHES

Roasted Pepper and Pasta Gratin

Servings: 8

A nice change from the usual pasta dishes. Dietary fiber: 11 grams.

1	pound whole-wheat penne or spiral pasta	1	bay leaf
3	tablespoons olive oil	¼	teaspoon salt
1	medium onion, chopped	½	teaspoon pepper, ground
4	garlic cloves, chopped	2	red peppers, roasted, peeled, and cut into ½-inch pieces (see p. 191)
1	28-ounce can low-sodium tomatoes, drained and chopped	2	green peppers, roasted, peeled, and cut into ½-inch pieces
1	15-ounce can tomato sauce	1½	cups 1% milk
1	teaspoon dried basil	1½	cups Parmesan cheese, grated
½	tablespoon dried thyme		

Preheat oven to 400° F.

Add pasta to a large pot of rapidly boiling water and stir. Cook until al dente (tender, but still firm). Drain and rinse with cold water. Toss with 1 tablespoon of olive oil.

Heat oil in large, heavy saucepan over medium heat. Add onion and cook until tender, about 6 minutes, stirring occasionally. Add garlic and sauté 2 minutes. Add drained chopped tomatoes and tomato sauce. Stir and add basil, thyme, bay leaf, salt, and pepper. Cook over medium heat for 15 minutes. Remove and discard bay leaf.

Spray an 8-cup baking dish with vegetable oil. Pour in ⅓ of the tomato sauce. Layer ⅓ of the pasta, ⅓ of the peppers, ⅓ of the milk, and ¼ of the cheese. Repeat twice. Sprinkle with remaining ¼ of cheese. Bake about 30 minutes or until top is browned and bubbly.

Serve hot with green beans or grilled eggplant or zucchini slices.

Per Serving: 390 Calories; 11g Fat (24.5% calories from fat); 18g Protein; 59g Carbohydrate; 14mg Cholesterol; 707mg Sodium. Exchanges: 3 Grain (Starch); 1 Lean Meat; 2½ Vegetable; 0 Nonfat Milk; 1½ Fat.

MAIN DISHES

Fettuccine with Broccoli Cheese Sauce

Servings: 4

*An easy way to convince kids to eat a super-healthy vegetable. Dietary fiber:
6 grams.*

8 ounces whole-wheat
    fettuccine pasta
2 cups broccoli florets with
    stems removed
2 tablespoons butter or
    margarine

2 tablespoons whole-wheat flour
2 cups 1% milk
⅔ cup part-skim ricotta cheese
½ cup grated Parmesan cheese
½ teaspoon salt
½ teaspoon freshly ground pepper

Cook pasta according to package directions. Drain and keep warm.

Break broccoli into small florets and cook in boiling water or steam until
tender (about 4 minutes). Drain and set aside.

Melt butter or margarine in medium saucepan. Add flour and cook, stirring constantly, for 1 minute. Slowly whisk in milk, stirring until blended.
Continue cooking, stirring constantly until sauce is thick, 10 to 15 minutes.
Add ricotta and Parmesan cheeses, salt, and pepper. Cook until well blended
and cheese is melted, about 5 minutes.

Spoon warm pasta into large serving bowl. Add broccoli cheese sauce
and stir to coat pasta, being careful not to break up broccoli florets.

*Per Serving: 427 Calories; 14g Fat (28.9% calories from fat); 23g Protein;
56g Carbohydrate; 41mg Cholesterol; 639mg Sodium. Exchanges: 3 Grain
(Starch); 1 Lean Meat; ½ Vegetable; ½ Nonfat Milk; 2 Fat.*

MAIN DISHES

Mushroom and Red Pepper Pasta

Servings: 4

Red peppers and balsamic vinegar give this quick and light pasta dish a tangy but subtle flavor. Dietary fiber: 8 grams.

8 ounces whole-wheat fusilli or penne cooked according to package directions	3 portobello mushroom caps, cleaned and sliced into ½-inch pieces
½ cup water, reserved from cooking pasta	1 tablespoon balsamic vinegar
2 tablespoons olive oil, divided	1½ teaspoons salt
½ cup chopped green onions	½ teaspoon freshly ground black pepper
1 large red pepper, chopped	8 ounces baby spinach leaves, washed and stems removed
2 garlic cloves, minced	

Toss pasta with 1 tablespoon of the olive oil. Keep warm.

In a medium skillet, heat the remaining tablespoon of olive oil. Add the green onions and red pepper and sauté, stirring often, until vegetables are tender, about 8 to 10 minutes.

Add the garlic and cook for 1 minute, stirring. Add mushrooms, vinegar, salt, and black pepper. Cook over medium heat until mushrooms are tender, about 8 minutes, stirring often.

Add spinach and reserved ½ cup water to mushroom mixture. Sauté, stirring to mix, until spinach is wilted, about 3 minutes.

Spoon warm pasta into large serving bowl. Stir mushroom mixture into pasta and toss, mixing to coat pasta.

Per Serving: 305 Calories; 8g Fat (22.2% calories from fat); 12g Protein; 52g Carbohydrate; 0mg Cholesterol; 844mg Sodium. Exchanges: 3 Grain (Starch); 2 Vegetable; 0 Fruit; 1½ Fat.

MAIN DISHES

Basmati Rice Jambalaya

Servings: 4

Raise the heat with more seasoning, or substitute seafood for sausage to alter this versatile Creole favorite. Dietary fiber: 2 grams.

1 cup uncooked basmati rice rinsed and drained	1 yellow bell pepper, chopped
1½ cups low-sodium chicken broth	1 small yellow onion, chopped
2 tablespoons butter or margarine	4 green onions, chopped
1 tablespoon olive oil	2 garlic cloves, minced
½ pound light smoked sausage (or turkey sausage)	1 tomato, seeded and chopped
1 red bell pepper, chopped	1 teaspoon Creole seasoning
	¼ teaspoon salt
	¼ teaspoon black pepper

Place rinsed basmati rice and chicken broth in medium saucepan. Bring to boil over medium-high heat, stirring occasionally. Let broth reduce to rice level, lower heat and cover with tight lid.

Simmer for 10 minutes or until broth is absorbed and rice is tender.

In a medium frying pan, melt butter and add olive oil. Add sliced sausage and brown over medium heat, stirring constantly. Add red and yellow peppers, yellow onions, green onions, garlic, and chopped tomato. Sauté for about 5 minutes or until vegetables are tender, stirring frequently. Stir in rice and Creole seasoning, salt and black pepper, mixing well. Heat thoroughly.

Variations: Cooked brown rice can be substituted for the basmati rice, which will add fiber to the dish. Remember that brown rice requires a longer cooking time than basmati rice, but it is well worth the effort.

Per Serving: 382 Calories; 18g Fat (42.2% calories from fat); 15g Protein; 42g Carbohydrate; 51mg Cholesterol; 813mg Sodium. Exchanges: 2 Grain (starch); 0 Lean Meat; 1½ Vegetable; 2 Fat; 0 Other Carbohydrates.

MAIN DISHES

Sweet Potato Chili

Servings: 6

A hearty, quick, meatless meal in one dish, extra high in fiber and flavor. Dietary fiber: 9 grams.

1	tablespoon olive oil	½	pound green beans, trimmed and cut in half
1	medium onion, chopped		
2	tablespoons chili powder	2	medium sweet potatoes, peeled and cut into ½-inch chunks
1	teaspoon ground cumin		
2	tablespoons chopped cilantro		
4	garlic cloves, chopped	1	teaspoon salt
1	jalapeño pepper, seeded and chopped	2	cups water
		1	15-ounce can black beans, rinsed and drained
1	28-ounce can diced tomatoes, undrained		

Heat oil in nonstick Dutch oven over medium heat until hot. Add onions and cook until tender, about 10 minutes. Stir occasionally.

Add chili powder, cumin, cilantro, garlic, and jalapeño, and cook 2 minutes while stirring. Add tomatoes and their juice, green beans, sweet potatoes, salt, and water. Heat over medium heat until boiling.

Reduce heat, cover and simmer for 35 to 45 minutes, until sweet potatoes and green beans are tender. Stir occasionally. Add drained black beans and heat through.

Per Serving: 182 Calories; 4g Fat (17.5% calories from fat); 7g Protein; 32g Carbohydrate; 0mg Cholesterol; 807mg Sodium. Exchanges: 1½ Grain (Starch); ½ Lean Meat; 2 Vegetable; ½ Fat.

MAIN DISHES

163

Red Beans and Brown Rice

Servings: 6

This is a traditional New Orleans dish, often served on Mondays. We eliminated the flour roux and substituted brown rice for white rice for a Sugar Buster version that is just as tasty and more nutritious. Dietary fiber: 22 grams.

1	pound dried red beans	½	cup chopped green bell pepper
½	pound ham cubes, for seasoning	1	bay leaf
2	quarts water	1	teaspoon ground red pepper
1½	cups chopped yellow onions	1	teaspoon Worcestershire sauce
3	garlic cloves, minced	3	cups cooked brown rice
1	cup chopped celery		(for basmati rice)

Rinse beans and place them in a saucepan. Add enough cool water to cover beans by 2 inches; bring to a boil and simmer for 2 minutes. Remove from heat, cover, and soak for 1 hour; drain. Discard the cooking liquid.

Place the soaked beans and ham in a large pot with a lid. Cover with water and bring to a boil.

Reduce heat to a simmer. Add all of the other ingredients and simmer partially covered for one hour or until beans are tender.

Remove ¾ cup of beans. Mash beans through a sieve into the pot. Spoon any remaining mashed beans into the pot. Remove and discard the bay leaf. Stir well to blend.

Serve over brown or basmati rice.

Per Serving: 690 Calories; 7g Fat (9.4% calories from fat); 32g Protein; 125g Carbohydrate; 22 mg Cholesterol; 557 mg Sodium. Exchanges: 8 Grain (Starch); 2 Lean Meat; 1 Vegetable; ½ Fat; 0 Other Carbohydrates.

MAIN DISHES

Quick Red Beans

Servings: 4

Cut the preparation and cooking time to less than thirty minutes without losing the flavor in this version of the classic red-bean dish. Dietary fiber: 10 grams.

2 tablespoons canola oil	1 10-ounce can Ro-Tel Diced
½ cup chopped onion	Tomatoes and Green
⅓ cup chopped celery	Chilies, or 1 10-ounce can
2 garlic cloves, minced	diced tomatoes, drained
1 tablespoon whole-wheat flour	2 15-ounce cans red kidney beans
	(New Orleans style), drained,
	reserving 1 cup liquid
	¼ teaspoon salt

Heat oil in a medium nonstick skillet over medium heat. Add onion, celery, and garlic and sauté, stirring frequently, until vegetables are soft, about 8 minutes.

Add whole-wheat flour, mixing well and stirring constantly for 1 minute. Add the drained tomatoes, red kidney beans, reserved liquid, and salt.

Cook for 10 minutes over low heat, stirring frequently to prevent sticking.

Serving Ideas: Serve over cooked brown or basmati rice, or as a side dish without rice.

Variation: Substitute canned navy or any other beans of your choice for a quick-cooking bean dish.

Per Serving: 198 Calories; 7g Fat (32.8% calories from fat); 8g Protein; 26g Carbohydrate; 0mg Cholesterol; 789 mg Sodium. Exchanges: 1½ Grain (Starch); ½ Lean Meat; ½ Vegetable; 1½ Fat.

MAIN DISHES

Black Bean Burritos

Servings: 4

Black beans with a kick and lots of fiber. Dietary fiber: 9 grams.

1	tablespoon olive oil	¼	teaspoon pepper
½	cup chopped onion	¼	teaspoon Creole seasoning
½	cup chopped green bell pepper	4	whole-wheat tortillas
3	garlic cloves, minced	4	ounces shredded Monterey Jack cheese
15	ounces canned black beans, rinsed and drained	1	cup shredded iceberg lettuce
¼	teaspoon salt	4	ounces tomato salsa

Spray nonstick medium skillet with cooking spray. Add olive oil and heat. Sauté onion, green pepper, and garlic over medium heat until tender, about 8 minutes.

Add beans, salt, pepper, and Creole seasoning to onion mixture. Mash some beans in pan to make mixture somewhat pasty. Heat thoroughly.

In a separate skillet, warm tortillas one by one or wrap tortillas in slightly moistened paper towels and heat in microwave.

Place 1 ounce of cheese on each whole-wheat tortilla and allow cheese to melt partially.

Spoon on lettuce and tomato salsa. Fold tortilla closed.

A dollop of sour cream can be added as an additional topping.

Per Serving: 487 Calories; 19g Fat (34.5% calories from fat); 20g Protein; 59g Carbohydrate; 25mg Cholesterol; 841mg Sodium. Exchanges: 3½ Grain (Starch); 1½ Lean Meat; ½ Vegetable; 3 Fat; 0 Other Carbohydrates.

Bagel Pizza

Servings: 4

Meal in a hurry! Dietary fiber: 1 gram.

2	2-ounce whole-wheat bagels, sliced in half	1	cup shredded mozzarella cheese
½	cup marinara sauce or any no-sugar-added pizza or tomato sauce	1	cup mushrooms, roasted bell peppers, or any other vegetable choice, sliced

Preheat oven to 350° F.

Top bagel halves with sauce, cheese, and vegetables and bake until cheese melts and crust is golden brown.

Per Serving: 190 Calories; 8g Fat (38.6% calories from fat); 10g Protein; 19g Carbohydrate; 25mg Cholesterol; 398mg Sodium. Exchanges: 1 Grain (Starch); 1 Lean Meat; 0 Vegetable; 1 Fat.

MAIN DISHES

Grilled Shrimp with Mango Salsa

Servings: 6

A light spring or summer meal that will delight the taste buds. Dietary fiber: 2 grams.

8 garlic cloves, thinly sliced
⅓ cup olive oil
   Juice of 2 limes (about
      2 tablespoons), divided
1 teaspoon salt
½ teaspoon pepper
2 pounds shrimp,
      shelled and deveined

2 ripe mangos, peeled and
      cut into chunks
1 small bunch green onions,
      white and light green parts
      only, thinly sliced on diagonal
2 jalapeños, seeded and finely diced
1 bunch cilantro, leaves only,
      chopped

In medium saucepan over low heat, cook sliced garlic in olive oil until soft. Add 1 tablespoon lime juice, salt, and pepper and let cool.

Put shrimp on 6 wooden skewers (soak skewers in water for 15 minutes to prevent burning). Place skewered shrimp in a long casserole dish and pour marinade over it, coating the shrimp well. Marinate in refrigerator for 2 to 6 hours.

Prepare salsa 30 minutes before serving; in a glass bowl mix the mangos, green onions, jalapeños, cilantro, and the remaining lime juice. Refrigerate until ready to serve.

Preheat a boiler or grill to high heat. Grill the skewered shrimp about 3 minutes on each side.

Serve the skewered shrimp on a bed of mango salsa.

Variation: Instead of grilling, sauté marinated and drained shrimp in 2 tablespoons of heated olive oil in a medium nonstick skillet on burner over medium-high heat for about 8 minutes until shrimp are cooked.

Serving Ideas: If shrimp is unavailable or your family prefers chicken, try grilling skinless deboned chicken breasts. Slice chicken into long slivers and serve over the mango salsa. Mango salsa is also a delicious accompaniment to grilled tuna.

Per Serving: 327 Calories; 15g Fat (40.6% calories from fat); 31g Protein; 17g Carbohydrate; 230mg Cholesterol; 583mg Sodium. Exchanges: 0 Grain (Starch); 4½ Lean Meat; ½ Vegetable; 1 Fruit; 2½ Fat.

MAIN DISHES

Shrimp and Couscous Salad

Servings: 4

A quick-cooking main-dish salad.

5¼ cups water, divided
  (4 cups and 1¼ cups)
1 pound medium shrimp
1 teaspoon celery seed
2 teaspoons salt
½ teaspoon cayenne pepper
1 cup uncooked couscous
¼ cup seasoned rice vinegar
2 teaspoons vegetable oil

1½ teaspoons soy sauce
½ teaspoon dark sesame oil
2 garlic cloves, chopped
1 cup shredded romaine lettuce
1 cup chopped red bell pepper
¼ cup chopped fresh cilantro
2 tablespoons finely chopped
    dry-roasted unsalted peanuts

Add celery seed, salt and cayenne pepper to four cups water in a medium saucepan. Bring to a boil and add shrimp, When the water begins to boil again cook the shrimp for about 3 minutes, remove the pan from the heat and allow the shrimp to soak for 10 minutes. Drain off the water and allow the shrimp to cool then, peel and devein the shrimp.

Bring 1¼ cups water to a boil in a saucepan, gradually stir in couscous. Remove from the heat; cover and let stand 5 minutes. Fluff with a fork; cool.

Combine vinegar, vegetable oil, soy sauce, sesame oil, and garlic in a large bowl, stir well. Add shrimp, couscous, lettuce, bell pepper and cilantro; toss well. Sprinkle with peanuts.

Serving Ideas: Serve with grilled or baked chicken or fish.

Per Serving: 355 Calories; 8g Fat (19.4% calories from fat); 30g Protein; 40g Carbohydrate; 173mg Cholesterol; 1380mg Sodium. Exchanges: 2½ Grain (Starch); 3½ Lean Meat; ½ Vegetable; 1 Fat; 0 Other Carbohydrates.

MAIN DISHES

Jazzy Shrimp Louisianne

Servings: 6

A well-seasoned spicy and flavorful dish. Dietary fiber: 7 grams.

2 tablespoons butter	2 slices lemon
¼ cup olive oil	1½ teaspoons salt
¼ teaspoon red pepper	1 teaspoon black pepper
½ teaspoon celery seed	2 pounds shrimp, shelled,
2 teaspoons dry mustard	deveined, and patted dry
½ teaspoon ginger	12 ounces cooked whole-wheat
2 teaspoons paprika	angel hair pasta, tossed with
⅛ teaspoon cardamom	2 tablespoons olive oil
1 bay leaf	

In a large skillet, melt the butter, then add the oil and mix well. Remove from heat.

Mix all the other ingredients except the shrimp and pasta in a small bowl. Add these ingredients to the oil. Mix well. Return the oil and spice mixture to burner and simmer over low heat for 5 minutes, stirring frequently. Remove the bay leaf and lemon slices and discard.

Add the peeled and dry shrimp to the skillet mixture and sauté over medium heat, stirring constantly until shrimp turn pink and are cooked, about 8 minutes.

Combine shrimp mixture and pasta, tossing well to coat pasta. Serve hot.

Serving Ideas: Serve shrimp over brown rice or basmati rice and sprinkle with chopped green onions.

Per Serving: 495 Calories; 17g Fat (30.5% calories from fat); 38g Protein; 47g Carbohydrate; 240mg Cholesterol; 801mg Sodium. Exchanges: 3 Grain (Starch); 4½ Lean Meat; 0 Vegetable; 0 Fruit; 3 Fat.

Oven-Fried Fish Filets

Servings: 4

Serve crispy fish without the fat from frying. Dietary fiber: 2 grams.

4 fish filets, firm fish of your choice (farm-raised catfish is perfect)

2 teaspoons Creole seasoning

¼ cup yellow mustard

1½ cups whole-wheat bread crumbs

1 teaspoon garlic powder

¼ teaspoon black pepper

Preheat oven to 350° F.

Wash fish filets and pat dry. Sprinkle with Creole seasoning. Rub each filet on all sides with enough yellow mustard to cover lightly. Set aside.

Combine breadcrumbs with garlic powder and black pepper on a large plate or sheet of wax paper and mix well. Dredge fish in crumbs. Place filets on a baking sheet that has been sprayed lightly with nonstick cooking spray and bake for 10 to 15 minutes or until fish is cooked through.

Per Serving: 368 Calories; 4g Fat (11.3% calories from fat); 47g Protein; 32g Carbohydrate; 99mg Cholesterol; 769mg Sodium. Exchanges: 2 Grain (Starch); 5½ Lean Meat; ½ Fat; 0 Other Carbohydrates.

MAIN DISHES

Grilled Salmon Asian Style

Servings: 4

A great source of omega-3 fatty acids, this salmon also packs lots of good taste. Dietary fiber: trace.

3 tablespoons olive oil	⅛ teaspoon garlic powder
2 tablespoons low-sodium soy sauce	¼ teaspoon cumin
2 tablespoons lemon juice	¼ teaspoon pepper
1 teaspoon dried rosemary	4 6-ounce salmon filets
3 teaspoons chopped fresh ginger	

Combine olive oil, soy sauce, lemon juice, rosemary, ginger, garlic, cumin, and pepper in a small bowl. Stir well. Divide the marinade in half. Coat the salmon filets on both sides with half of the marinade; reserve the other half. Marinate the filets for ½ hour.

Preheat grill to medium. Grill filets 6 to 8 minutes on each side. Place salmon on serving platter and spoon reserved marinade on top.

Per Serving: 296 Calories; 16g Fat (49.8% calories from fat); 34g Protein; 2g Carbohydrate; 88mg Cholesterol; 415mg Sodium. Exchanges: 0 Grain (Starch); 5 Lean Meat; 0 Vegetable; 0 Fruit; 2 Fat.

MAIN DISHES

Side Dishes

Vegetable Medley

Servings: 6

An unusual and colorful veggie combination. Dietary fiber: 4 grams.

1	large sweet potato, peeled and cut into ½-inch slices	1	tablespoon olive oil
1	medium eggplant, cut into ½-inch cubes	2	tablespoons balsamic vinegar
1	large green pepper, cut into ½-inch slices	1	teaspoon lemon juice
		2	garlic cloves, minced
		1	teaspoon dried basil leaves
1	large onion, cut into ½-inch slices	1	teaspoon dried oregano
1	large tomato, cut into 6 wedges	1	teaspoon salt
		¼	teaspoon pepper

Preheat oven to 400° F.

Line a flat baking sheet with foil and spray with cooking spray. Place sliced vegetables in single layer on pan and spray them with cooking spray.

Bake for 30 minutes or until vegetables are tender. Remove vegetables from oven and place them in a medium bowl.

While vegetables are cooking, combine olive oil, vinegar, lemon juice, garlic, basil, oregano, salt, and pepper in a small bowl. Stir well. Pour dressing over vegetables and toss to coat.

Serving Ideas: Can be served as a vegetable or spooned into pita pockets for a meal in one dish.

Per Serving: 83 Calories; 3g Fat (26.3% calories from fat); 2g Protein; 15g Carbohydrate; 0mg Cholesterol; 363mg Sodium. Exchanges: ½ Grain (Starch); 1½ Vegetable; 0 Fruit; ½ Fat.

SIDE DISHES

Eggplant Dressing

Servings: 6

This is an appetizing dish that can be served as a vegetable casserole or baked under chicken pieces as a low-glycemic, low-fat dressing. Dietary fiber: 5 grams.

2 medium eggplants, peeled and cut into ¼-inch chunks	1 tablespoon Worcestershire sauce
Salt and pepper to taste	2 tablespoons olive oil
1 cup chicken broth	1 medium onion, chopped
3 slices whole-wheat bread, diced	½ cup chopped celery
½ teaspoon Italian seasoning	4 garlic cloves, chopped

Place eggplant in a medium glass bowl. Sprinkle lightly with salt and pepper, toss well, and set aside.

In a medium bowl, soak bread chunks in chicken broth. Add Italian seasoning and Worcestershire sauce, stirring well and mashing bread with a fork until mixture is smooth. Set aside.

Heat olive oil over medium heat in a large nonstick skillet. Add onion, celery, and garlic. Cook for 6 minutes or until vegetables are tender, stirring often with a wooden spoon.

Add eggplant to skillet and mix well. Cook over medium-low heat for 5 minutes, stirring often.

Add chicken broth and bread mixture to skillet; mix thoroughly. Cook over medium heat for 25 minutes or until eggplant is tender. Stir and scrape the bottom of the pan frequently to prevent sticking. Additional amounts of chicken broth can be added 2 tablespoons at a time if sticking occurs.

Serving Idea: Eggplant mixture can be added, after it has cooked for about 10 minutes, to a baked chicken dish midway through the oven cooking: Bake 6 skinless seasoned chicken pieces in large, covered, shallow baking pan at 350° F for 40 minutes. Remove chicken baking dish from oven. Move chicken pieces to perimeter of dish. Spoon partially cooked eggplant mixture in center, covering with chicken pieces. Cover mixture with dish lid or foil. Return to oven and bake additional 20 to 30 minutes or until chicken is done.

Per Serving: 133 Calories; 6g Fat (35.4% calories from fat); 4g Protein; 19g Carbohydrate; trace Cholesterol; 233mg Sodium. Exchanges: ½ Grain (Starch); 0 Lean Meat; 2½ Vegetable; 1 Fat; 0 Other Carbohydrates.

SIDE DISHES

Eggplant Parmigian

Servings: 6

Eliminate the breading and frying of eggplant for a dish that is as good as the traditional one but that is healthier and easier to prepare. Dietary fiber: 7 grams.

2 medium eggplants	⅔ cup grated Parmesan cheese
5 cups Basic Tomato Sauce (page 157)	Salt and pepper to taste
½ pound provolone cheese slices	

Preheat oven to 350° F.

Peel eggplants and slice into ½-inch ovals. Rinse and drain eggplant slices. Salt and pepper eggplant and set aside.

Spray a 9 × 12–inch rectangular glass baking dish with cooking spray. Cover the bottom of the dish with 1½ cups of the tomato sauce.

Place a layer of sliced eggplant over the sauce. Place single slices of provolone cheese over the eggplant and sprinkle with ½ of the Parmesan cheese. Cover with 1½ cups of tomato sauce.

Add remaining eggplant slices and cover with additional provolone slices and Parmesan cheese. Top with remaining tomato sauce.

Cover dish with aluminum foil and bake for 30 to 45 minutes until eggplant is fork-tender. Uncover and continue to bake for 10 to 15 minutes to reduce the amount of liquid.

Per Serving: 330 Calories; 20g Fat (53.0% calories from fat); 17g Protein; 23g Carbohydrate; 33mg Cholesterol; 1047mg Sodium. Exchanges: 0 Grain (Starch); 1½ Lean Meat; 4 Vegetable; 2½ Fat.

SIDE DISHES

Creole Okra

Servings: 4

A spicy change from the usual vegetable side dish. Dietary fiber: 5 grams.

1 pound fresh or frozen okra, sliced thin	3 garlic cloves, minced
2 tablespoons olive oil	1 14-ounce can Ro-Tel diced tomatoes
1 medium onion, chopped	1 teaspoon salt
½ green bell pepper, chopped	¼ teaspoon black pepper

If fresh okra is used, wash and dry the okra and slice each piece thin. If frozen okra is used, defrost the okra until all pieces are separated.

In a heavy medium skillet, heat oil and sauté okra for about 10 minutes, stirring frequently. Add bell pepper, onions, and garlic, sautéing until tender, about 5 minutes.

Add diced tomatoes with liquid, salt, and pepper. Cover and simmer over low heat, stirring frequently until okra is tender, about 20 minutes, depending on whether okra is fresh or frozen.

Per Serving: 140 Calories; 7g Fat (44.1% calories from fat); 4g Protein; 17g Carbohydrate; 0mg Cholesterol; 552mg Sodium. Exchanges: 0 Grain (Starch); 3 Vegetable; 1½ Fat.

Zucchini Stir-Fry

Servings: 4

A quick vegetable sauté that is a good accompaniment to any entrée. Dietary fiber: 2 grams.

2 tablespoons olive oil	4 medium zucchini
1 tablespoon unsalted butter or margarine	½ teaspoon salt
	½ teaspoon red pepper flakes
1 small yellow onion, chopped	

Cut zucchini into 6-inch-long julienne strips.

Heat the olive oil and butter in a medium skillet over low heat. Add the chopped onion and sauté for 3 minutes.

Raise the heat to medium, add the zucchini, salt, and red pepper flakes. Sauté, tossing frequently, until zucchini is tender but slightly crisp, about 5 minutes. Serve hot.

Per Serving: 123 Calories; 10g Fat (67.7% calories from fat); 3g Protein; 8g Carbohydrate; 8mg Cholesterol; 274mg Sodium. Exchanges: 0 Grain (Starch); 1½ Vegetable; 2 Fat.

SIDE DISHES

Zucchini Bolognese

Servings: 8

A vegetable casserole with all the flavor of lasagne but without the noodles. Dietary fiber: 4 grams.

4	large zucchini	1	teaspoon salt
2	medium onions, sliced	1	teaspoon oregano
3	Italian sausage links	1	teaspoon garlic powder
¾	cup water	1	teaspoon pepper
1	8-ounce package shredded part-skim mozzarella cheese	1	28-ounce can puréed tomatoes
		½	cup part-skim ricotta cheese
½	pound mushrooms, sliced		

Trim zucchini; cut into thin lengthwise slices with a sharp knife.

Place onion slices and Italian sausages in a large skillet with water; cook over medium heat, stirring often, until water evaporates; then stirring constantly until onion slices are golden. Remove from heat. When sausages are cool, remove casing from sausage and discard; chop sausages.

Layer one-third of the zucchini slices in an 8-cup shallow casserole. In casserole, combine shredded mozzarella cheese with mushrooms. Top zucchini with part of the cheese and mushroom slices. Combine salt, oregano, garlic powder, and pepper in a cup. Sprinkle part of the spices over the zucchini. Layer with one-third of the onion meat mixture and tomatoes. Repeat to make three layers, each sprinkled with remaining spice mixture.

Cover with aluminum foil.

Bake in moderate oven, 350° F, for 40 minutes. Remove foil and bake uncovered 20 minutes longer, or until zucchini is tender and casserole is bubbly. Zucchini produces water when cooked; spoon off excess liquid if necessary. Spoon ricotta cheese on top and let stand 10 minutes before serving.

Serving Idea: This hearty dish can be served as an entrée with a broccoli or green bean salad.

Per Serving: 260 Calories; 17g Fat (58.6% calories from fat); 15g Protein; 13g Carbohydrate; 45mg Cholesterol; 823mg Sodium. Exchanges: 0 Grain (Starch); 1½ Lean Meat; 2 Vegetable; 2½ Fat.

SIDE DISHES

Stuffed Bell Peppers

Servings: 10

A well-seasoned combination. Substitute cooked brown rice for the basmati for additional fiber and a heartier dish. Dietary fiber: 3 grams.

10	medium green bell peppers	1	teaspoon freshly ground
2	pounds lean ground beef		black pepper
1½	cups chopped onion	¼	teaspoon cayenne pepper
2	tablespoons canola oil	1	28-ounce can tomatoes,
2	tablespoons minced parsley		drained and chopped
1	tablespoon finely chopped garlic	3	cups cooked basmati rice
1	teaspoon dried thyme	2	tablespoons Worcestershire sauce
1	teaspoon dried basil	1	cup grated Parmesan cheese
2	teaspoons salt		

Slice off tops of green peppers. Remove seeds and membranes and wash peppers under cold water.

Drain and set aside.

In a large, heavy skillet, heat the oil over medium heat. Sauté onions and ground beef until the beef is brown and cooked.

Add parsley, garlic, thyme, basil, salt, black pepper, and cayenne pepper. Cook for about 5 minutes, stirring frequently. Add the tomatoes to the mixture, continuing to stir. Cook for 3 minutes. Add the cooked rice and Worcestershire sauce and mix well. Cover skillet and cook over low heat for 5 minutes.

Remove skillet from the heat and stir in the grated cheese. Stuff the peppers with rice mixture.

Place the stuffed peppers in a 9 × 12–inch glass baking dish to which 1 inch of hot water has been added. Cover the pan with foil and cook for 45 minutes, or until peppers are tender.

When the peppers are cooked, remove foil and allow tops to brown (about 5 to 10 minutes longer).

Serving Idea: Serve with steamed or sautéed vegetables and a large green salad.

Per Serving: 546 Calories; 25g Fat (42% calories from fat); 26g Protein; 53g Carbohydrate; 74mg Cholesterol; 825mg Sodium. Exchanges: 2½ Grain (Starch); 3 Lean Meat; 2½ Vegetable; 3 Fat; 0 Other Carbohydrates.

SIDE DISHES

Spinach Artichoke Pie

Servings: 6

Who said kids won't eat spinach? Dietary fiber: 5 grams.

2   packages frozen spinach
3   tablespoons margarine
4   tablespoons chopped leeks
1   10½-ounce can mushroom soup
1   14-ounce can artichoke hearts,
     drained and chopped

2   tablespoons grated Parmesan
     cheese
½   teaspoon salt
¼   teaspoon black pepper
¼   teaspoon Tabasco sauce
3   large eggs, beaten

Preheat oven to 350° F.

Cook spinach according to package directions; remove from heat and drain well, pressing out all liquid with a fork.

In a medium saucepan, melt the margarine over medium heat. Add chopped leeks and sauté until tender.

Add drained spinach, mushroom soup, artichoke hearts, Parmesan cheese, salt, pepper, and Tabasco sauce. Mix well.

Remove from heat and cool slightly. Add beaten eggs to spinach mixture, stirring quickly to blend eggs thoroughly.

Spray a glass pie plate with vegetable oil. Add spinach mixture.

Bake for 30 minutes or until pie is set.

Cut into wedges and serve.

Serving Idea: Serve with lean grilled chicken, meat, or fish and tossed green salad.

Variation: Green onions can be used instead of leeks.

Per Serving: 155 Calories; 10g Fat (53.4% calories from fat); 7g Protein; 12g Carbohydrate; 64mg Cholesterol; 575mg Sodium. Exchanges: 0 Grain (Starch); ½ Lean Meat; 2 Vegetable; 1½ Fat.

SIDE DISHES

Spicy Sweet Potato Gratin

Servings: 4

For those who like spicy foods, this is a different way to prepare sweet potatoes. Dietary fiber: 3 grams.

1 cup 1% milk	Salt and pepper to taste
½ cup sugar-free maple syrup	3 leeks, white part only,
3 garlic cloves, chopped	sliced thin
1 Ancho chile, seeded and chopped	½ cup shredded Monterey Jack
2 large sweet potatoes, peeled and	cheese
sliced thin	

Preheat oven to 350° F.

Lightly spray a medium-sized casserole dish with vegetable spray.

In a small saucepan, heat the milk and maple syrup. Remove the mixture from the heat, add the garlic and chopped chile, and let steep for 30 minutes.

Purée the milk mixture in a blender or food processor.

Lay one-third of the sweet potato slices in the casserole dish, overlapping slightly. Season with salt and pepper.

Ladle one-third of the milk mixture over the sweet potatoes. Sprinkle with one-third of the leeks and one-third of the cheese.

Repeat the layering two more times, seasoning each layer of sweet potatoes lightly with salt and pepper.

Cover with foil and bake for 40 minutes. Uncover and bake for another 20 minutes or until brown and bubbly. Remove from oven and let sit for 10 minutes.

Per Serving: 294 Calories; 5g Fat (16.1% calories from fat); 8g Protein; 55g Carbohydrate; 15mg Cholesterol; 132mg Sodium. Exchanges: 1 Grain (Starch); ½ Lean Meat; 2 Vegetable; 0 Nonfat Milk; ½ Fat; 2 Other Carbohydrates.

SIDE DISHES

Sweet Potato Frisbees

Servings: 4

A much better fry, both in taste and nutrition. Dietary fiber: 2 grams.

3   tablespoons unsweetened
      orange juice
2   teaspoons canola oil
½   teaspoon ground ginger
½   teaspoon salt

¼   teaspoon ground red pepper
2   large sweet potatoes,
      peeled and sliced into
      ¼-inch-thick slices

Preheat oven to 350° F.

In a small saucepan, combine the orange juice, canola oil, ground ginger, salt, and red pepper. Bring mixture to a boil; reduce heat and simmer for 3 minutes. Remove from heat and let cool.

Combine sweet potato slices and juice mixture in a large bowl; mix well. Drain sweet potatoes.

Spray baking sheet with nonstick spray. Arrange sweet potatoes in a single layer on the baking sheet and bake for 30 minutes.

Per Serving: 94 Calories, 2g Fat (23.6% calories from fat); 1g Protein; 17g Carbohydrate; 0mg Cholesterol; 275mg Sodium. Exchange: 1 Grain (Starch); 0 Vegetable; 0 Fruit; ½ Fat.

SIDE DISHES

Spicy Lentils

Servings: 10

A *delicious high-fiber, low-glycemic dish. Dietary fiber: 10 grams.*

1 pound dried lentils	¼ cup extra-virgin olive oil
1 quart water	1 10-ounce can Ro-Tel Diced
2 teaspoons salt	Tomatoes and Chilies,
1 medium onion, chopped	drained

Rinse and drain lentils in colander.

Cover lentils with 1 quart water; add salt and simmer in covered pan until tender, about 45 minutes.

Check pan frequently and add water if needed.

In a small skillet sauté the onion in olive oil until tender.

Add onion, olive oil, and tomatoes to the lentils, stirring carefully.

Cook for 10 to 15 minutes.

Serving Idea: Can be served over brown rice for added fiber. Save leftover lentils for preparation of Italian Lentil Soup.

Per Serving: 210 Calories; 6g Fat (24.4% calories from fat); 13g Protein; 28g Carbohydrate; 0mg Cholesterol; 518mg Sodium. Exchanges: 1½ Grain (Starch); 1 Lean Meat; 0 Vegetable; 1 Fat.

SIDE DISHES

183

Green Beans and Onions

Servings: 4

Low in calories, high in fiber—crisp, fresh green beans, simply prepared, are a wholesome addition to any meal. Dietary fiber: 4 grams.

1 pound fresh green beans,
   washed, ends snapped off,
   and cut in half
2 chicken bouillon cubes
1 medium yellow onion, chopped

¼ teaspoon freshly ground
    black pepper
1 tablespoon melted butter
    or margarine

Bring 4 cups water to boil in a medium pan; add bouillon cubes and beans. Reduce the heat and add chopped onion.

Bring beans to a simmer and cook partially covered, until barely tender, about 20 minutes.

Drain; add salt, pepper, and melted butter. Serve hot.

Variation: For a nutritious salad, rinse green beans, toss with one sliced, roasted red pepper and one sliced, roasted yellow pepper. Combine 2 tablespoons olive oil, 1 tablespoon white wine vinegar and 2 teaspoons Dijon mustard. Pour over bean mixture, toss well to coat beans, and marinate for 1 hour.

Per Serving: 73 Calories; 3g Fat (37.4% calories from fat); 3g Protein; 10g Carbohydrate; 8mg Cholesterol; 408mg Sodium. Exchanges: 0 Grain (Starch); 0 Lean Meat; 2 Vegetable; ½ Fat.

SIDE DISHES

Snacks

Pita Triangles

Servings: 4

Serve these crispy pita chips with tomato salsa or another nutritious dip of your choice. Dietary fiber: 3 grams.

2 6-inch whole-wheat pita breads
4 teaspoons olive oil
2 teaspoons dried oregano (optional)

4 tablespoons grated Parmesan
    cheese (optional)

Preheat broiler with oven rack 5 inches from heat.

Cut each pita in half horizontally and place rough side up on an ungreased baking sheet.

Spread 1 teaspoon of olive oil on each pita half and sprinkle each half with ½ teaspoon of oregano and 1 tablespoon of Parmesan cheese.

Cut each pita slice into 6 wedges with a sharp knife or kitchen shears.

Broil until the cheese is melted and the edges are lightly browned, about 2 minutes. Watch closely to prevent burning.

Serve immediately or, when cooled, cover and refrigerate for later use. Chips can be reheated in a 350° F oven, but are best when prepared just before serving.

Per Serving: 150 Calories; 7g Fat (39.8% calories from fat); 5g Protein; 18g Carbohydrate; 4mg Cholesterol; 263mg Sodium. Exchanges: 1 Grain (Starch); ½ Lean Meat; 1 Fat.

SNACKS

Crostini with Olives and Sun-Dried Tomatoes

Servings: 8

Richly flavored appetizer or snack. Dietary fiber: 2 grams.

8	whole-wheat French baguette slices	¼	cup chopped, pitted black olives
4	ounces sun-dried tomatoes	3	ounces reduced-fat cream cheese
2	garlic cloves, minced	4	ounces feta cheese
		2	tablespoons 1% milk

Preheat oven to 300° F.

Arrange slices of whole-wheat bread on baking sheets. Bake for 6 minutes. Turn slices over, bake 6 minutes or until golden brown.

Finely chop tomatoes. Place tomatoes in medium bowl. Stir in garlic and chopped olives. Set aside.

Beat cream cheese until softened. Beat in feta and milk until smooth. To serve, spread cheese mixture on crostini slices. Top with small dollop of tomato mixture.

Per Serving: 93 Calories; 4g Fat (37.9% calories from fat); 4g Protein; 11g Carbohydrate; 12mg Cholesterol; 420mg Sodium. Exchanges: ½ Grain (Starch); ½ Lean Meat; 0 Vegetable; 0 Fruit; 0 Nonfat Milk; ½ Fat; 0 Other Carbohydrates.

Tomato Salsa

Yield: 2 cups

Prepare when good ripe summer tomatoes are available as a dip for whole-wheat toasted rounds or as a delicious accompaniment to taco salad, pitas, chicken, or fish. Dietary fiber: 1 gram.

4	large plum tomatoes	1	teaspoon chopped jalapeño pepper
¼	cup chopped green onions	1	tablespoon olive oil
¼	cup chopped cilantro	3	teaspoons lime juice
2	garlic cloves, minced		Salt and freshly ground
1	tablespoon chopped fresh oregano		black pepper to taste

Cut tomatoes in half lengthwise and remove seeds. Chop the tomatoes and place them in a glass bowl.

Add the remaining ingredients to the tomatoes. Allow flavors to blend at room temperature for about 10 minutes. Serve immediately or refrigerate and serve within 3 hours.

Per Serving: 35 Calories; 2g Fat (57% calories from fat); 1g Protein; 3g Carbohydrate; 0mg Cholesterol; 7mg Sodium. Exchanges: 0 Grain (Starch); 0 Lean Meat; ½ Vegetable; 0 Fruit; ½ Fat.

SNACKS

Salmon Party Ball

Servings: 8

A great-tasting salad or party appetizer that provides nutritious fatty omega-3 oils. Dietary fiber: 1 gram.

16 ounces canned salmon	1 teaspoon prepared horseradish
8 ounces Philadelphia Light cream cheese	¼ teaspoon salt
	½ cup chopped pecans
1 tablespoon lemon juice	3 tablespoons snipped parsley
2 teaspoons grated onion	

Drain and flake salmon. In a medium bowl, combine salmon, cream cheese, lemon juice, onion, horseradish, and salt. Mix well.

Chill salmon mixture for several hours.

Combine pecans and parsley on sheet of wax paper. Shape salmon mixture into a ball and roll the salmon in the nut mixture.

Serving Idea: Serve with whole-wheat crackers, or omit the pecans and parsley and spoon salmon mixture onto lettuce leaves for a nutritious lunch salad.

Per Serving: 172 Calories; 12g Fat (58.3% calories from fat); 15g Protein; 4g Carbohydrate; 39mg Cholesterol; 266mg Sodium. Exchanges: 0 Grain (Starch); 2 Lean Meat; 0 Vegetable; 0 Fruit; 1½ Fat; 0 Other Carbohydrates.

SNACKS

Spinach Artichoke Dip

Servings: 10

A creamy dip perfect for an appetizer or party. Dietary fiber: 4 grams.

20 ounces frozen chopped spinach
2 tablespoons butter or margarine
1 small onion, chopped fine
8 ounces Philadelphia Light
   Cream Cheese
8 ounces light sour cream

½ teaspoon salt
½ teaspoon Tabasco sauce
1 14-ounce can artichoke hearts,
   drained and chopped fine
½ cup grated Parmesan cheese

Prepare frozen spinach according to package directions. Drain well in a colander, pressing out all liquid with a fork. Set aside.

Melt butter or margarine in a medium nonstick skillet. Add chopped onion and sauté over low heat until onion is tender, about 5 minutes.

Add cream cheese and cook over low heat, stirring constantly until cheese is smooth. Add sour cream, salt, Tabasco sauce, and artichoke hearts. Mix well after each ingredient is added. Stir in Parmesan cheese. Heat through. Serve hot.

Serving Idea: Serve with whole-wheat crackers or toasted pita triangles.

Per Serving: 131 Calories; 8g Fat (51.1% calories from fat); 8g Protein; 10g Carbohydrate; 19mg Cholesterol; 422mg Sodium. Exchanges: ½ Lean Meat; 1½ Vegetable; 1 Fat; 0 Other Carbohydrates.

SNACKS

Caponata

Servings: 10

A fantastic snack, appetizer, salad, or side dish. Keeps several weeks in refrigerator, with flavor improving over time. Dietary fiber: 6 grams.

2 medium eggplants	⅓ cup red wine vinegar
½ cup extra-virgin olive oil	2 teaspoons salt
2 large onions, chopped	2 tablespoons dried basil
1½ cups celery, sliced ½ inch thick	4 tablespoons tomato paste
2 bell peppers, red or green, cut into 1-inch chunks	½ cup chopped parsley
2 garlic cloves, chopped	1 teaspoon freshly ground black pepper
2½ pounds tomatoes, seeded and diced	¾ cup sliced stuffed green olives
	4 tablespoons capers (optional)

Cut unpeeled eggplant into 1-inch cubes. Heat olive oil in a 5- or 6-quart nonreactive dutch oven. Add eggplant and onions and sauté for 5 minutes until lightly golden.

Add remaining ingredients to casserole; mix gently but thoroughly and simmer covered for 30 minutes, stirring occasionally. Remove lid and simmer for 10 minutes more or until thick. This will depend on the juiciness of the tomatoes. Serve at room temperature in a bowl surrounded by toasted whole-wheat bread rounds or whole-wheat crackers. Or serve as a salad on romaine leaves.

Per Serving: 182 Calories; 13g Fat (57.5% calories from fat); 3g Protein; 18g Carbohydrate; 0mg Cholesterol; 629mg Sodium. Exchanges: 0 Grain (Starch); 3 Vegetable; 0 Fruit; 2½ Fat; 0 Other Carbohydrates.

Roasted Bell Peppers

Servings: 6

Prepare large batches of this nutritious and delicious vegetable to add color and flavor to salads, pastas, and pitas. Dietary fiber: 1 gram.

2	red bell peppers	2	green bell peppers
2	yellow bell peppers	2	teaspoons olive oil

Trim tops and bottoms off the peppers and discard. Slice peppers in half and cut away the seeds and core.

Preheat the broiler and place the peppers skin side up 3 to 4 inches from the heat. Check peppers frequently, and broil until the skin blackens all over.

Place the broiled peppers in a paper or plastic bag and let stand for 10 minutes. Remove them from the bag and peel off the skin. Slice the peppers in thin strips; drizzle with olive oil. Place peppers in a glass jar or bowl and if not used immediately, refrigerate covered until ready to use.

Serving Idea: Toss peppers with cooked penne wheat pasta. Add Italian salad dressing. Chill, then serve as pasta salad.

Per Serving: 45 Calories; 2g Fat (30.9% calories from fat); 1g Protein; 8g Carbohydrate; 0mg Cholesterol; 2mg Sodium. Exchanges: 1½ Vegetable; ½ Fat.

SNACKS

Dip for Vegetables

Servings: 6

It will be easy to convince your family to eat raw veggies if you serve them with this easy-to-prepare dip. Dietary fiber: 3 grams.

8	ounces light sour cream	3	cups broccoli florets
1	package Good Seasons Zesty Italian Salad Dressing Mix	3	cups cauliflower florets
		3	stalks celery, julienned

Place sour cream in a small glass bowl. Add packet of salad dressing mix. Stir well. Place on a serving tray surrounded by cut vegetables.

Per serving: 46 Calories; 1g Fat (16.3% calories from fat); 3g Protein; 8g Carbohydrate; 3mg Cholesterol; 478mg Sodium. Exchanges: 0 Lean Meat; 1 Vegetable; 0 Fat; 0 Other Carbohydrates.

Hummus

Servings: 8

Perfect dip for pita triangles. Dietary fiber: 3 grams.

1	15-ounce can chickpeas, drained	½	teaspoon salt
¼	cup tahini	½	teaspoon ground cumin
3	tablespoons lemon juice	1	tablespoon olive oil
1	garlic clove, minced	½	teaspoon chopped fresh parsley
½	teaspoon cayenne pepper		

In a food processor or blender, combine chickpeas, tahini, lemon juice, garlic, cayenne pepper, salt, cumin. Process until smooth. Spoon the hummus onto a dish and smooth out the surface. Drizzle the olive oil over the hummus and garnish with the parsley.

Per Serving: 126 Calories; 6g Fat (43.9% calories from fat); 4g Protein; 14g Carbohydrate; 0mg Cholesterol; 301mg Sodium. Exchanges: 1 Grain (Starch); 0 Lean Meat; 0 Vegetable; 0 Fruit; 1 Fat.

SNACKS

Sugar Busters Ice Cream Float

Servings: 1

An easy and delicious treat. Add fruit for variety.

½ cup Sugar Busters! Vanilla   1   cup 1% milk
     Ice Cream or other ice cream   2   ice cubes
     with no added sugar

Scoop ice cream into blender or food processor. Add milk and ice cubes. Process until smooth.

Serving Ideas: Purée ½ pint fresh strawberries or ½ cup sliced mangos, peaches, or berries. Add ice cream and milk and blend well.

Per Serving: 192 Calories; 8g Fat (33.0% calories from fat); 11g Protein; 24g Carbohydrate; 30mg Cholesterol; 189mg Sodium. Exchanges: 1 Nonfat Milk; ½ Fat.

SNACKS

Tofu Shake

Servings: 4

Dietary fiber: 1 gram.

12	ounces firm tofu (Mori-Nu brand)	5	ice cubes
1	cup strawberries	1	packet non-caloric sweetener
½	cup no-sugar-added orange juice		

Place tofu, strawberries, and orange juice in blender or food processor and blend until mixed. Add ice cubes and sweetener. Blend until mixture is uniform.

Per Serving: 91 Calories; 4g Fat (36.4% calories from fat); 7g Protein; 8g Carbohydrate; 0mg Cholesterol; 8mg Sodium. Exchanges: 0 Grain (Starch); 2 Lean Meat; ½ Fruit; ½ Fat.

SNACKS

Trail Mix

Servings: 4

Dietary fiber: 14 grams.

2   cups bran cereal
1   ounce peanuts (about 20 peanuts) or any other nuts
2   ounces dried fruit

Toss cereal, nuts, and dried fruit into a Ziploc bag.
   Shake and enjoy.

Per Serving: 137 Calories; 5g Fat (23.2% calories from fat); 7g Protein; 29g Carbohydrate; 0mg Cholesterol; 4mg Sodium. Exchanges: 1½ Grain (Starch); 0 Lean Meat; ½ Fruit; 1 Fat.

Whole-Wheat Pizza

Servings: 6

Add your favorite toppings to an easily prepared pizza dough. Dietary fiber: 6 grams.

2½ cups whole-wheat bread flour   2   tablespoons olive oil
1   packet rapid-rise yeast   1   teaspoon salt
1   cup warm water

Preheat oven to 400° F.

In medium bowl, stir rapid-rise yeast into whole-wheat bread flour. Mix well.

Heat water and olive oil in small saucepan to 120° to 130° F.

Slowly stir water and oil into flour mixture. Stir until dough forms a ball; cover dough with a dishtowel and put in warm place for 10 to 15 minutes.

Oil rolling pin lightly with olive oil. Roll out dough into a 12- to 15-inch circle.

Place pizza on pan or stone and top with tomato sauce and cheese.

Bake for 20 minutes.

Per Serving: 213 Calories; 5g Fat (21.9% calories from fat); 7g Protein; 37g Carbohydrate; 0mg Cholesterol; 360mg Sodium. Exchanges: 2½ Grain (Starch); 0 Lean Meat; 1 Fat.

SNACKS

Whole-Wheat Crepes

Servings: 8

Crepes can be used with seafood, meat, or chicken fillings for a meal in one dish, or filled with fruit and light cream cheese for a dessert following a light salad entrée. Dietary fiber: 3 grams.

1½ cups whole-wheat flour	¾ cup water
3 eggs	¼ teaspoon salt
¾ cup 1% milk	1 tablespoon vegetable oil

Combine the whole-wheat flour, eggs, milk, water, salt, and vegetable oil in a blender and mix for 30 seconds. Scrape down the sides of the blender and process until smooth, another 30 seconds. Refrigerate batter for about an hour so that the crepes will be light in texture.

Coat a 10-inch crepe pan or nonstick skillet with cooking spray and place the pan over medium heat until just hot.

Pour 3 tablespoons of the batter into the pan, tilting pan quickly so that the batter covers the pan. Cook about 30 seconds. When crepe can be loosened from pan, flip it or turn with a spatula. Cook for about 30 seconds. This side will be just spotty brown and will be the side on which the filling is placed. Repeat until all of the batter is used.

When crepes are cool, stack between layers of waxed paper to prevent sticking.

Per Serving: 125 Calories; 4g Fat (27.8% calories from fat); 6g Protein; 18g Carbohydrate; 71mg Cholesterol; 101mg Sodium. Exchanges: 1 Grain (Starch); ½ Lean Meat; 0 Nonfat Milk; ½ Fat.

SNACKS

Gelatin Gigglers

Servings: 4

Dietary fiber: 1 gram.

1 envelope unsweetened gelatin powder
2 cups unsweetened apple juice

Add apple juice to gelatin powder and stir.
  Pour mixture into pint-sized shallow pan.
  Refrigerate for 4 hours.
  Gelatin may be cut using cookie cutters.

Yield: 4 ½-cup servings

Per Serving: 64 Calories; trace Fat (1.9% calories from fat); 2g Protein; 14g Car-bohydrate; 0mg Cholesterol; 7mg Sodium. Exchanges: 0 Lean Meat; 1 Fruit.

Fruit Dip

Servings: 6

Surround this delicious dip with low-glycemic sliced fruit. Dietary fiber: 2 grams.

1 cup fresh strawberries	1 packet Splenda or other
¼ cup unsweetened applesauce	non-caloric sweetener
1 cup low-fat, no-sugar-added	(optional)
vanilla yogurt	

Wash and trim strawberries. Chop fine.

In a medium bowl, mix strawberries, applesauce, yogurt, and Splenda. Chill.

Per Serving (excluding unknown items): 44 Calories; 1g Fat (11.1% calories from fat); 2g Protein; 8g Carbohydrate; 2mg Cholesterol; 25mg Sodium. Exchanges: 0 Fruit; 0 Fat; ½ Other Carbohydrates.

SNACKS

Frozen Fruit Delight

Servings: 9

Lots of calcium and fruit make this a healthy snack, salad, or dessert. Dietary fiber trace.

8 ounces Philadelphia Light Cream Cheese	1 envelope gelatin powder
	2 tablespoons mayonnaise
1 15-ounce can no-sugar-added fruit cocktail in juice, drained and with ½ cup liquid reserved	8 ounces low-fat no-sugar-added vanilla yogurt
	3 packets Splenda or other non-caloric sweetener
1 tablespoon lemon juice	

In small bowl, soften cream cheese in microwave for about 45 seconds; stir.

Drain fruit cocktail, reserving ½ cup of juice.

Set fruit aside. Mix reserved juice with lemon juice.

Sprinkle gelatin over juice mixture, stir to dissolve and let set 1 minute.

Combine softened cream cheese, mayonnaise, yogurt, and non-caloric sweetener. Stir well.

Fold fruit into cream cheese mixture.

Heat gelatin mixture. Do not boil.

Add gelatin mixture to cream cheese and fruit, stirring well to mix.

Pour into 8 × 8–inch shallow Pyrex dish, cover with foil and freeze until set; no longer than 2 hours. Remove from freezer to refrigerator until ready to serve.

With sharp knife, cut three rows down and three rows across to make 9 servings.

Serving Ideas: Serve over lettuce leaves as a salad or top with fresh fruit slices of your choice for garnish.

Per Serving: 155 Calories; 7g Fat (40.3% calories from fat); 5g Protein; 20g Carbohydrate; 11mg Cholesterol; 202mg Sodium. Exchanges: ½ Lean Meat; ½ Fruit; 1 Fat; 1 Other Carbohydrates.

SNACKS

18

Frequently Asked Questions

Many parents included questions they have about the Sugar Busters lifestyle in the comment section of our research survey. We have answered many questions during Sugar Busters presentations, in media interviews, and have also reviewed questions from our Web site so we have an idea of what you want to know. We hope that we have answered many of your questions in the text of this book, but include the following most frequently asked questions.

Q. Is the Sugar Busters way of eating good for children?
A. Yes, Sugar Busters is based on consumption of low-glycemic carbohydrates, lean and trimmed meats, high-fiber vegetables, whole grains, and fruit. It includes avoidance of added sugar, high-fat, over-processed foods, and fast foods. Adoption of this lifestyle will help children maintain a normal weight and decrease the risk of diabetes, hypertension, and vascular diseases later in life. Could any other way of eating be healthier?
Q. Is there research on a low-glycemic carbohydrate diet in children?
A. Yes, Dr. David Ludwig at Children's Hospital in Boston studied 107 obese children during a four-month period. Children in the study on the low-glycemic carbohydrate diet experienced a signifi-

cantly greater weight loss compared with those on the standard reduced-fat diet.

Q. Doesn't the body need a certain amount of added sugar each day?

A. No. Any sugar needed by the body can come from ingested carbohydrates such as fruits, beans, and wheat bread. The body does not need added sugar.

Q. My child participates in sports, in particular, long-distance running. Does Sugar Busters provide all that is needed for vigorous activity?

A. Low-glycemic carbohydrates are excellent sources of energy for athletes. During and immediately after a long-distance race, sports drinks containing water, electrolytes, and low to moderate amounts of sugar can be consumed to rapidly replenish the glycogen utilized during strenuous activity.

Q. How can I get my child to eat vegetables?

A. Different textures appeal to different children. Raw vegetables appeal to some children, while al dente (slightly firm) or well-cooked vegetables may appeal to others. So offer lots of variety and vary your presentation methods. Remember to continue to reintroduce vegetables even if they are rejected. Use flavorful seasonings. Simple preparation is healthier, but if all else fails serve vegetables with **small** amounts of sauce made from stone-ground wheat flour, low-fat milk, and low-fat cheeses. Have a variety of colorful fresh vegetables stored in the refrigerator always ready as finger foods to be served with low-fat, nutritious dips.

Q. Are artificial sweeteners safe for children?

A. After much research, there is no scientific evidence to indicate that artificial sweeteners are harmful. However, some patients have complained of headaches, muscle aches, and joint pains that have resolved when they discontinued use of artificial sweeteners. Yes, we consider them safe. Use them in moderation. Our recommendation for children is a maximum of 2 diet drinks per day.

Q. Since fructose has a low-glycemic index, would high-fructose corn syrup be an acceptable sweetener?

A. No, because high-fructose corn syrup is 50% fructose and 50% glucose, and that raises the glycemic index equal to sucrose or table sugar.

Q. What can my child eat on special occasions and at birthday parties?

A. We see no problem with occasional consumption of cake and ice cream for special events. Desserts should not be eaten regularly.

Q. May I have fruit with meals?

A. Yes. Eating fruit with meals may cause indigestion or "heartburn" for some people. However, if you do not have this problem, fruit may be eaten with a meal.

Q. Can I use Splenda?

A. Splenda is an excellent sugar substitute with minimal caloric value and no health hazard.

Q. Why are carrots not okay?

A. Carrots are a root vegetable with a high glycemic index of approximately 70. Beta-carotene, which is the pigment giving carrots their color and which is important for vitamin A synthesis, can be obtained by eating sweet potatoes, squash, and broccoli, all lower-glycemic carbohydrates. Small amounts of carrots can be added to soups, stews, salads, or crudités to garnish or add color.

Glossary

Amino acids. The building blocks of proteins, there are nine essential amino acids that the body cannot manufacture and that have to be obtained from foods.

Antioxidant. A substance that prevents the addition of oxygen in a chemical reaction and may retard the aging process. Vitamins A, C, and E are antioxidants.

Arteriosclerosis. A process associated with aging characterized by plaque formation inside arteries (blood vessels).

Body Mass Index (BMI). A calculation based on the weight and height of a person, it is a better assessment of the presence or absence of obesity than other methods.

Calorie. The unit of heat required to raise the temperature of water to one degree Celsius.

Carbohydrates. A class of a major food group that includes sugars and starches. Typically they contain only carbon, oxygen, and hydrogen. Carbohydrates are stored in the liver and muscles as glycogen, the storage form of sugar.

Cholesterol. A compound belonging to a family of substances called sterols, which combine with fats and circulate in the bloodstream.

Complex carbohydrates. A carbohydrate with multiple molecules of sugar (glucose) attached by chemical bonds.

Diabetes mellitus (Type 1). A disease characterized by lack of insulin and most commonly seen in young people, also called juvenile diabetes. Lack of insulin causes very elevated blood sugar levels and may cause acidosis.

Diabetes mellitus (Type 2). A disease characterized by resistance of the cells to the actions of insulin, also resulting in elevated blood-sugar levels. It is most common in obese adults.

Disaccharides. Sugars containing two simple sugar molecules attached by a bond, examples are fructose and lactose.

Fats. A class name of a major food group that includes oils and animal fats. Fats are made up of fatty acids.

Fatty acids. The chemical component of fat. Some are nutritionally essential.

Fiber. A non-digestible component of complex carbohydrates. Fiber can be insoluble (does not dissolve in water) or soluble. A high-fiber diet is considered to be a healthy diet.

Fructose. A simple sugar commonly found in fruits and vegetables, it has a modest glycemic index.

Glucagon. Hormone secreted by the pancreas that helps regulate blood sugar and also helps metabolize stored fat.

Glucose. The form in which sugar circulates in the bloodstream, it is the body's main source of energy.

Glycemic index. A term used to describe a carbohydrate's ability to raise the blood sugar over a period of time after ingestion.

Glycemic load. A measurement of the effect of an ingested carbohydrate on blood sugar. The amount of the carbohydrate and its glycemic index are used in a formula to obtain the glycemic load (number of grams of the carbohydrate multiplied by the glycemic index).

Glycogen. A complex form of glucose, which is stored in the body and used to meet energy needs between meals.

HDL Cholesterol. The form of cholesterol circulating in the bloodstream in the form of high-density lipoproteins, thought to be protective against heart disease.

Hypoglycemia. The term for low blood sugar. Reactive hypoglycemia can occur several hours after the ingestion of high-glycemic carbohydrates. Spontaneous hypoglycemia can occur with the use of some medications, in association with certain tumors, and in dysfunction of some endocrine organs.

Insulin. A hormone secreted by the pancreas that controls blood sugar and influences protein synthesis and fat metabolism.

Junk food. Generally made of high-glycemic carbohydrates and combined with fat. Easily recognizable because it is generally contained in cellophane or other plastic wrappers and is inexpensive.

Lactose. A disaccharide sugar, which is found in milk, it has a modest glycemic index.

LDL cholesterol. The form of cholesterol circulating in the bloodstream in the form of low-density lipoproteins; high levels are thought to be a major risk factor for heart disease.

Lipolysis. The breakdown of stored fat into component fatty acids. This chemical reaction is inhibited by high-circulating insulin levels.

Monounsaturated fats. Fat molecules which contain only one double bond and are therefore better fats; examples are olive and canola oils.

Obesity. The presence of excess body fat, best determined by calculating Body Mass Index.

Omega-3 fatty acids. Fat found in fish, which has been found to have health benefits such as the lowering of cholesterol.

Phytochemicals. Chemicals that are derived from plants. Many of these have health benefits.

Proteins. A class name of a major food group that includes animal proteins (meats) and vegetable proteins (beans, lentils). Proteins are composed of amino acids and are the building blocks of the body.

Refined grains. Grains which have been milled and processed by removing the bran or outer layer. Most of the fiber and nutrients are removed during this process and the glycemic index is high. An example is refined wheat flour.

Saturated fat. Fat molecules whose carbon atoms are fully saturated with hydrogen atoms. This type of fat is generally found in animals, is thought to be less desirable, and should be restricted in the diet.

Glossary

Simple sugars. One-molecule sugars. Examples are glucose, fructose, and galactose.

Sucrose. A disaccharide sugar commonly found in table sugar.

Whole grains. Grains that have been only partially milled or processed, thus retaining nutrients and fiber and having a lower glycemic index. An example is stone-ground wheat flour.

References

Attwood CW. Obesity trends and genes. *www.vegsource.com/attwood/obesity.htm* 2000.

Berenson G.S., Srinivasan S.R., Nicklas T.A. "Atheroscelerosis: a Nutritional Disease of Childhood." *Am J Cardiol* (1998) Nov 26;82(10B):22T–29T.

Blumenthal J.A., Babyak M.A., Moore K.A. "Effects of Exercise Training on Older Patients with Major Depression." *Arch Intern Med* (1999) Oct 25;159(19):2349–56.

Chatenoud L., Vecchia C.L. et al. "Refined-Cereal Intake and Risk of Selected Cancers in Italy." *Am J Clin Nutr* (1999) 70:1107–10.

Cruz J.A. "Dietary Habits and Nutritional Status in Adolescents Over Europe—Southern Europe." *Eur J Clin Nutr* (2000) Mar;54 Suppl 1:S29–35.

Diamond F.B. "Newer Aspects of the Pathophysiology, Evaluation, and Management of Obesity in Childhood." *Current Opinion in Pediatrics* (1998);10:422–427.

Diamond, Jared. *Guns, Germs, and Steel.* New York: Norton, 1998. p97,125.

Dietz W.H. *American Academy of Pediatrics Guide to Your Child's Nutrition.* (New York: Villard, 1999), p45.

Ding Z, HE Q, Fan Z. "National epidemiological study on obesity of

References

children aged 0–7 years in China 1996." *Chung Hua I Hsueh Tsa Chih* (1998) Feb;78(2):121–23.

Donath S.M. "Who's Overweight? Comparison of the Medical Definition and Community Views." *Med J Aus* (2000) Apr17;172(8):375–7.

Dwyer, J. "Should Dietary Fat Recommendations for Children Be Changed?" *J Am Diet Assoc* (2000) Jan;100(1): 36–37.

Heini, A.F., Weinsier, R.L. "Divergent Trends in Obesity and Fat Intake Patterns: the American Paradox." *Am J Med* (1997): Mar;102:259–264.

Foster-Powell, K. Brand-Miller, J. "International Tables of Glycemic Index." *Am J Clin Nutr* (1995);62:871S–93S.

Freedman, D.S., Dietz, W.H., Srinivasan, S.R., Berenson G.S., et al. "The Relationship of Overweight To Cardiovascular Risk Factors Among Children and Adolescents: the Bogalusa Heart Study." *Pediatrics* (1999):Jun;103(6 Pt 1):1175–82.

Gordon-Larsen, P., McMurray, R.G., Popkin, B.M. "Determinants of Adolescent Physical Activity and Inactivity Patterns." *Pediatrics* (2000) Jun;105(6): 1e83.

Guthrie, J.F., Morton, J.F. "Food Sources of Added Sweeteners in the Diets of Americans." *J Am Diet Assoc* (2000):100:43–48, 51

Guyton, A.C., Hall, J.E. *Textbook of Medical Physiology 10th Edition.* Philadelphia: W.B. Saunders Co., 2000. p785–786.

Hudgins, L.C., Hellerstein, M.K., Seidman, C.E., et al. "Relationship Between Carbohydrate-Induced Hypertriglyceridemia and Fatty Acid Synthesis in Lean and Obese Subjects." *J Lipid Research* (2000);41:595–604.

Jacobs, D.R., Meyer, K.A., Kushi, L.H., et al. "Whole-Grain Intake May Reduce the Risk of Ischemic Heart Disease Death in Postmenopausal Women: the Iowa Women's Health Study." *Am J Clin Nutr* (1998);68:248–57.

Jacobsen, M.F. "Liquid Candy: How Soft Drinks are Harming American's Health." www.cspinet.org/sodapop/liquid_candy.htm 2000.

Jenkins, D.J.A., et al. "Glycemic Index of Foods: A Physiological Basis for Carbohydrate Exchange." *Am J Clin Nutr* (1981);34:362–66.

Kaufman, M. "Fighting the Cola Wars in Schools." *Washington Post,* March 23, 1999, p. Z12.

Levi, F., Pasche, C., et al. "Refined and Whole Grain Cereals and the Risk of Oral, Oesophageal and Laryngeal Cancer." *Eur J Clin Nutr* (2000) Jun;54(6):487–9.

Salmeron, J., Manson, J.E., Stampfer, M.J. et al. "Dietary Fiber, Glycemic Load, and Risk of Non-Insulin-Dependent Diabetes Mellitus in Women." *JAMA* (1997) Feb;277(6):472–77.

Sheslow, D., Hassink, S., Wallace, W., DeLancey, E. "The Relationship Between Self-Esteem and Depression in Obese Children." *Ann NY Acad Sci* (1993) Oct 29;699:289–91.

Spieth, L.E., Harnish, J.D., Ludwig, D.S., et al. A Low-Glycemic Index Diet in the Treatment of Pediatric Obesity." *Arch Pediatr Adolesc Med* (2000) Sep;154(9):947–51.

Spiller, G.A., ed. *CRC Handbook of Dietary Fiber in Human Nutrition, 2nd Edition.* (Boca Raton: CRC Press, 1992).

Steward, H.L., Bethea, M.C., Andrews, S.S., Balart, L.A. *Sugar Busters! Cut Sugar to Trim Fat.* (New York: Ballantine Books, 1998).

Wee, S.L., Williams, C., Gray, S., Horabin, J. "Influence of High and Low Glycemic Index Meals on Endurance Running Capacity." *Med Sci Sports Exerc* (1999) Mar;31(3):393–99.

Weisburger, J.H. "Evaluation of the Evidence on the Role of Tomato Products in Disease Prevention." *Proc Soc Exp Biol Med* (1998) Jun;218(2):140–3.

Willi, S.M., Oexmann, J., Wright, N.M., et al. "The Effects of High-Protein, Low-Fat, Ketogenic Diet on Adolescents with Morbid Obesity: Body Composition, Blood Chemistries, and Sleep Abnormalities." *Pediatrics* (1998);101:61–67.

Wildey, M.B., Pampalone, S.Z., Pelletiere, R.L. "Fat and Sugar Levels are High in Snacks Purchased from Student Stores in Middle Schools." *J Am Diet Assoc* (2000) Mar;100(3):319–22.

Williams, D.E., Knowler, W.C., Smith, C.J., et al. "Indian or Anglo Dietary Preferences and the Incidence of Diabetes in Pima Indians." *Diabetes* (2000) May;49 Suppl 1:A39.

Wolever, T.M.S., Jenkins, D.J.A., Jenkins, A.L., Josse, R.G. "The Glycemic Index: Methodology and Clinical Implications." *Am J Clin Nutr* (1991);54:846–54.

References

Liu, S., Stampfer, M.J., Hu F.B., et al. "Whole-Grain Consumption and Risk of Coronary Heart Disease: Results from the Nurses' Health Study." *Am J Clin Nutr* (1999) Sep;70(3):412–19.

Lowry, R., Galuska, D.A., Fulton, J.E., et al. "Physical Activity, Food Choice, and Weight Management Goals and Practices Among U.S. College Students." *Am J Prev Med* (2000) Jan;18(1):18–27.

Ludwig, D.S., Majzoub, J.A., Al-Zahrani, A., et al. "High Glycemic Index Foods, Overeating, and Obesity." *Pediatrics* (1999):Mar;103(3):E26.

Martinez, J.A. "Obesity in Young Europeans: Genetic and Environmental Influences." *Eur J Clin Nutr* (2000):Mar;54 Suppl 1:S56–60.

McMurray, R.G., Bauman, M.J., Harrell, J.S., et al. "Effects of Improvement in Aerobic Power on Resting Insulin and Glucose Concentrations in Children." *Eur J Appl Physiol* (2000) Jan;81(1–2):132–39.

Meyers, A.F., Sampson, A.E., Weitzman, M., et al. "School Breakfast Program and School Performance." *Am J Dis Child* (1989) Oct;143(100):1234–39.

Must, A., Jacques, P.F., Dallad, G.E., et al. "Long-Term Morbidity and Mortality of Overweight Adolescents. A follow-up of the Harvard Growth Study of 1922 to 1935." *New Eng J Med* (1992): 327:1350–355.

Noriega, E., Rivera, L., Peralta, E. "Glycemic and Insulinaemic Indices of Mexican Foods High in Complex Carbohydrates." *Diabetes Nutr Metab* (2000) Feb;13(1):13–19.

Ohlson, M.A., Hart, B.P. Influence of breakfast on total day's food intake. *J Am Diet Assoc* (1965);47:282–86.

Popkin, B.M., Udry, J.R. "Adolescent Obesity Increases Significantly in Second and Third Generation U.S. Immigrants: The National Longitudinal Study of Adolescent Health." *J Nutr* (1998) Apr; 128(4):701–6.

Salmeron, J., Ascherio, A., et al. "Dietary Fiber, Glycemic Load, and Risk of NIDDM in Men." *Diabetes Care* (1997) Apr;20(4):545–50.

Index

213

Index

RHYMES FOR KIDS

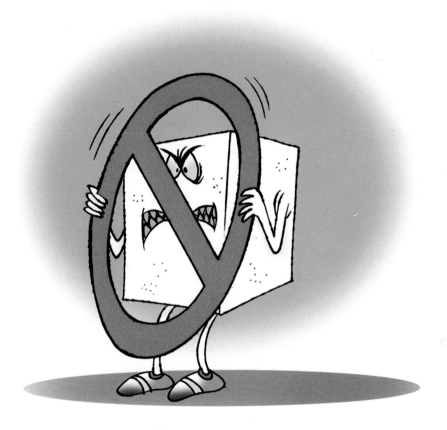

Written by Linda Andrews
Illustrated by Walt Handelsman

Letter to Kids

Dear Kids,

    This is a letter from the Sugar Busters authors right to you. You are a unique person. This means that there is no one just like you on the face of the earth. You go to school to learn and prepare for a bright and successful future. Just as an athlete trains for a race or a tournament, you must prepare and get your body ready for learning, growth, and development. You can do this with the help of your parents and by making the right food choices.

    Just as car needs the right fuel—gasoline—to run just right, so does your body need the right fuel—food—to give you energy and nutrients to grow strong and healthy. Learning about foods and nutrition can be boring, so we want you to learn, in a fun way, which foods are best for you and which foods you should stay away from.

    It would be great if you could stop making bad food choices in one day. That is hard. It probably won't happen in a day or even a few weeks. But if you make changes little by little, you won't miss the foods that are not so good for you and you will start getting used to—and even like—the foods that are good for you. It is like meeting a new friend. The more time you spend with the friend, the more you feel good about being with him or her.

    The journey to eating healthy food can be a lot of fun. It takes some learning and some deter-mination. But this book will help you and your parents learn about good food choices and show you ways to stick with those choices.

What may be hard is that you will see all of those fun commercials on TV for foods that are not good for you. Guess what? Just because a food is on TV doesn't mean that it is good for you or that you should eat it.

Why is it important to be a Sugar Buster? Would you put sand in your car to make it run? No way! Sand will fill up your tank, but it certainly won't help your car to run, and it will take up space so that there will be no room for the good fuel. Just a little sugar is needed for your body, but if you put too much in, it takes up the space that healthy foods need to have. We believe that too much sugar adds fat to your body. Sugar can add too much weight and be unhealthy.

There are some foods that quickly turn into sugar after you eat them. These foods, such as white potatoes (especially french fries), candy, and soft drinks can be unhealthy. If you stay away from these foods that some kids eat too often, and switch them with foods that are good for you, then you will be on the right track. You will have a good start as a Sugar Buster who is eating to make a strong and healthy body.

We wrote a book for adults first. The grown-ups liked the book. One person told another person about how the book helped them and it went on and on. We know that kids need the same kind of help. Read on and learn how to be a Sugar Busters Kid.

Good Luck with Good Nutrition,
The Sugar Busters Authors

Stop, look, and listen to these tales we have to tell
By the end of the story, you will know Sugar Busters well.
Now our story is a tale of very good WOE
Way Of Eating we call it and we want you to know
That eating this way is the right way to grow.
Journey with the Sugar Busters Kids to learn some facts,
About very healthy meals and wholesome snacks.
If you think learning about food is boring and bland,
We'll spice up this story and add a brass band.

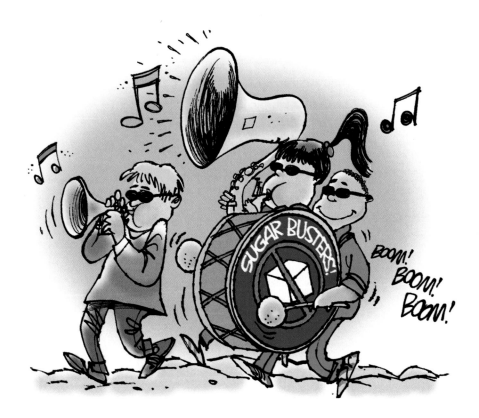

Sugar Buster is the detective who will help us find
The hidden healthful benefits in foods of all kinds.
A body that is lean, active, and strong,
Will give you a life that is healthy and long.

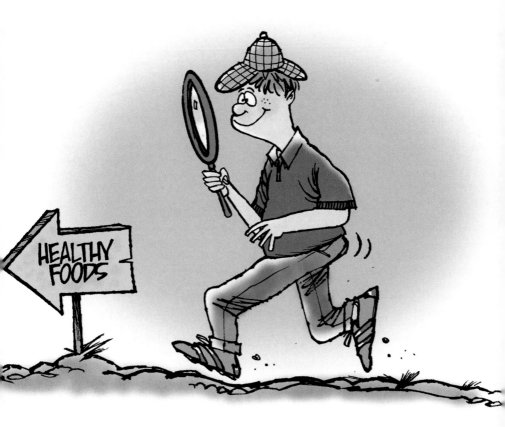

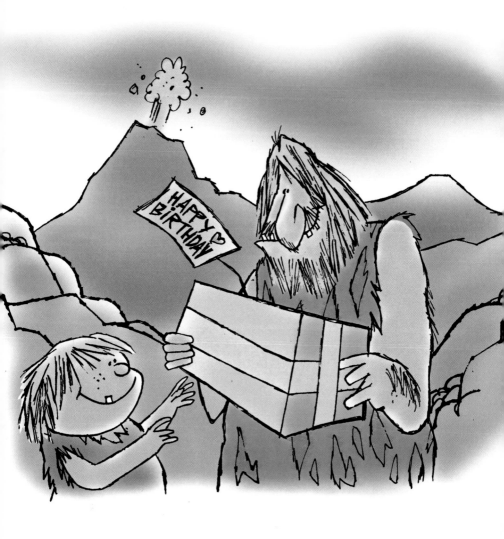

There was a time when our ancestors roamed the earth
(Well, it was a very long time before your birth)
That there was no sugar, not even for birthday cakes
And everyone ate healthier food, for gosh sakes!
No french fries, soft drinks, or candy,
Food was more natural when fast food wasn't handy.

Sugar is the mean villain in this tale of good nutrition
'Cause we want to keep our bodies healthy and in the
    best condition.
Sugar can't help us. It will just add pounds.
So avoid it often, and that is not as bad as it sounds.
Don't eat candy or cake as a snack
'Cause it will quickly get you off the right track.
Instead pick the right kind of fruit for snacks,
And fill them to the brim of your backpacks.
Eat lots of apples, oranges, pears, and plums,
Grapes, mangos, and kiwis, so many to choose from.

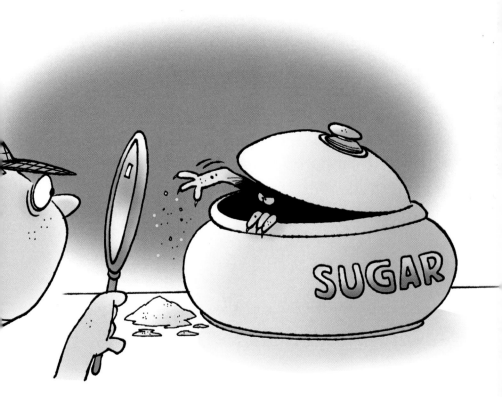

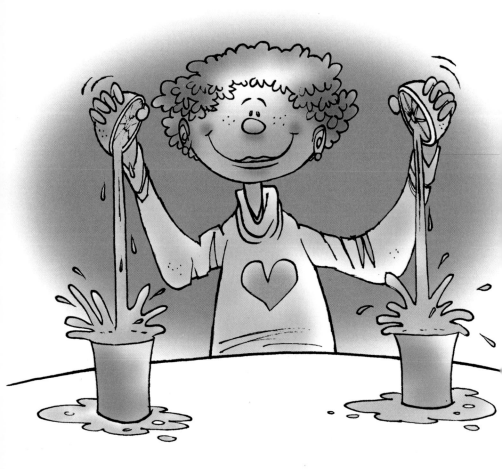

Now there is hidden sugar that we need to know about,
So read the food labels to scout the villain out.
Some fruit drinks you think are really good for you
Are loaded with sugar, and we know there are quite a few.
It's better to get your nutrition from the fruit itself,
Be sure to read the label on the drink before you
    take it from the shelf.
Pure fruit juice with no sugar added is what you want.
Why not squeeze it yourself and cut down on the hunt?

A mill is a place where grain is processed into food to eat,
And one of the healthiest foods there is made from wheat.
Researchers have found, and it is surprising,
That before we make the bread and set it aside for rising,
The wheat grain used must NOT be so refined
That the healthy part is removed and left behind.

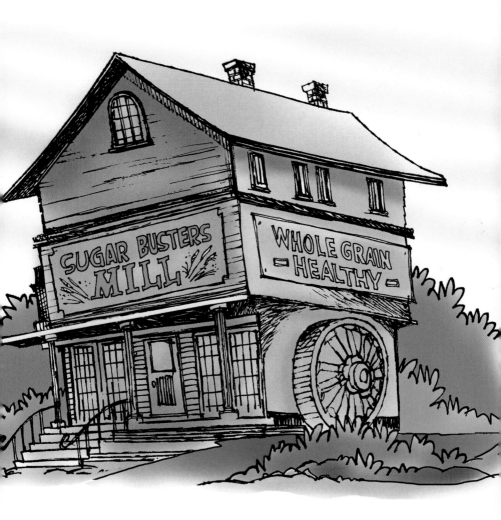

So we can forget mushy and hard-to-swallow
    bread that is white.
Instead eat whole-wheat bread and enjoy every bite.
Multigrain, rye, and barley breads are all okay,
Serve up a pita pocket and get your fiber for today.
The same is true of pasta, be it long, short, or round.
Whole-wheat pasta is so much better for you,
Just spoon on some sauce and serve up a mound.

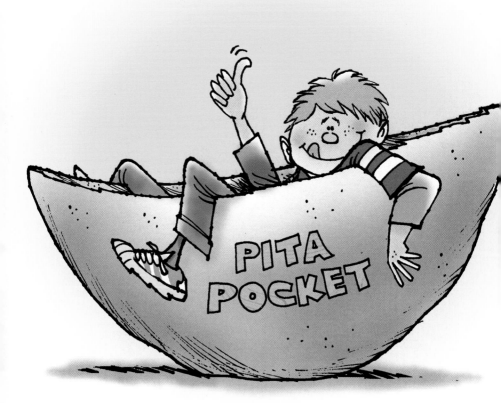

PITA
POCKET

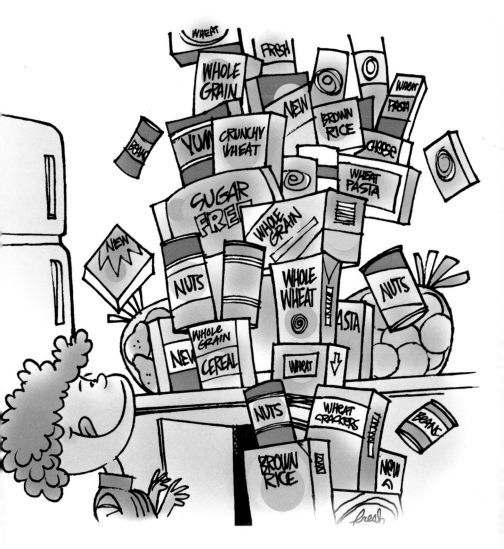

Yesterday Kari raided kitchen cabinets and the
    refrigerator door
She separated fare that she didn't want anymore.
The number of Sugar Busters foods was piled so high
That they reached to the attic, past the roof,
    and into the sky.
Eating this way, she thought, won't be so hard,
And a fit and healthy body will be her reward.

Cheese is okay, but don't eat too much,
And remember, candy is something you shouldn't touch.
Oh my! Now what is there to drink?
This is something that really makes you think:
Soda pop is full of sugar with no nutritional value of note.
So bathing all those organs with crystal-clear water gets
    our vote.
Low-fat milk, that great teeth-and-bone strengthener,
Is our choice for the perfect body lengthener.
What we mean is, of course, you know:
Milk helps all of the body's bones to grow.

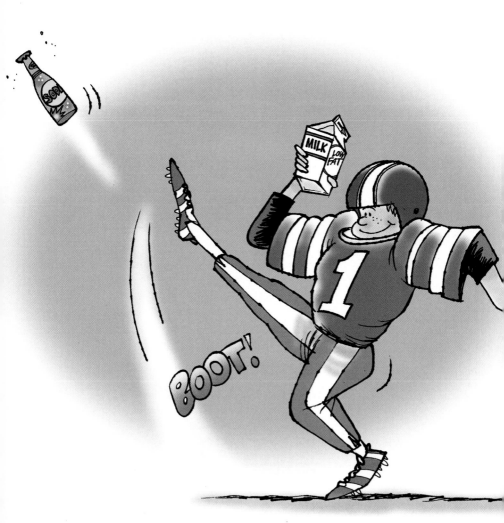

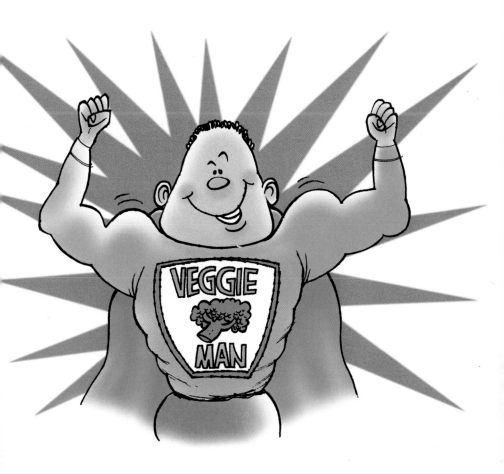

Veggies, veggies, why do they give you a scare?
We will give you and Mom some recipes to prepare.
They can be quite delicious when cooked with the
    right seasoning.
Eat them often and we know you will agree with our reasoning.
Because they give you vitamins, minerals, and
    disease prevention,
They are really one of the healthiest foods that
    we can mention.
So broccoli, spinach, and cauliflower are not food to scorn,
But a true Sugar Buster would forget the french
    fries and corn.

Where oh where have all the kids gone?
They used to be pitching ball out on the lawn.
Instead at home in front of the TV they can be found.
Before, they used to be running to reach the baseball mound.
Video games and TV just can't take the place
Of a good old-fashioned neighborhood race.
"I'd rather just sit and watch them play," you say,
No! Get out there and exercise each and every day.
So turn off the TV and get off of your duff,
'Cause most kids today just don't exercise enough.

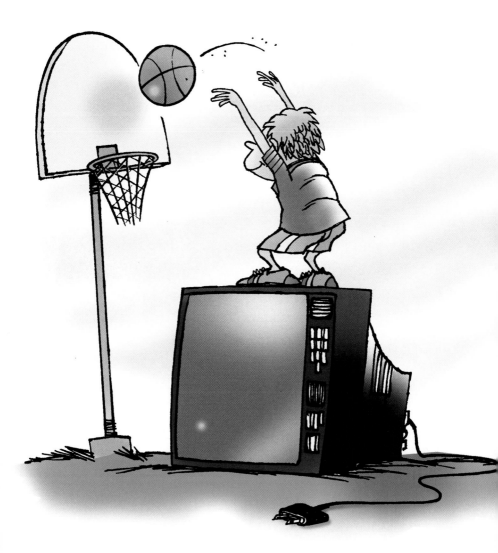

Beans, beans, yes, by all means.
In any shape or color we need beans.
Black, red, green, or white (often called navy)
Simmered with seasonings in water, will make their own gravy.
Beans, beans, as tall as Jack's stalk they can sprout
If I can't get them down here I'll climb to the top to
　　shake them out.

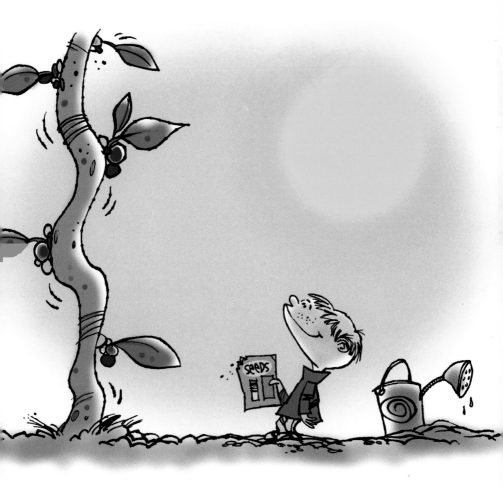

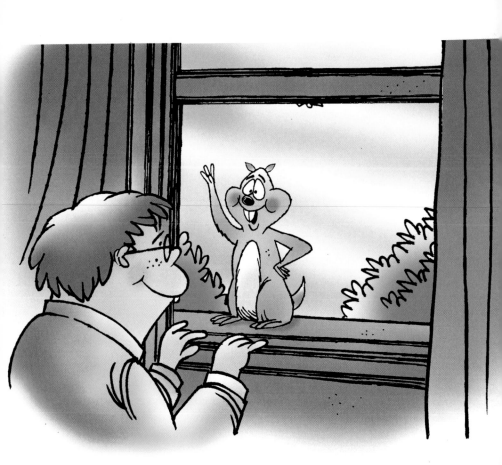

Eating, eating, munching away,
Timothy sat in front of the TV all day.
And as the house got stuffier and stuffier,
His cheeks got puffier and puffier.
A chipmunk observing from a nearby tree,
Peered in and said, "why, he looks just like me!"
The problem that poor Timothy didn't see
Was that the chipmunk's food was as healthy as could be.
Acorns and nuts and natural things like that,
Were better than potato chips fried in fat.

You won't see chipmunks eating sugary donuts and such.
They would rather be scurrying about than
     sitting around watching TV so much.
The reason animals are so trim and alert
Is that they eat the right foods and have more energy
     to exert.

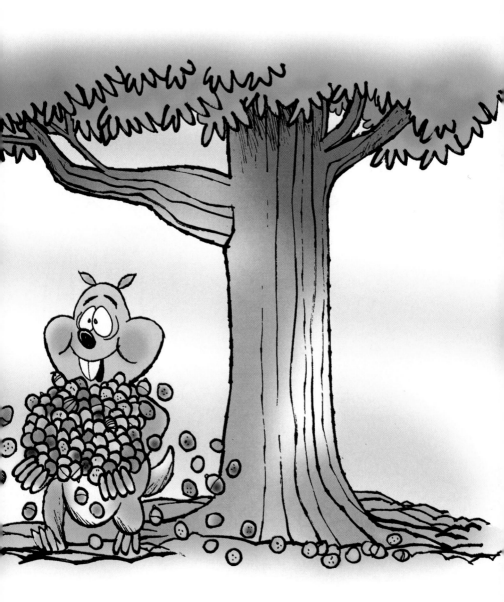

Berries, berries everywhere!
I'm covered with berries so let me climb on to a chair
If there are any more berries around
Heaven knows I will surely drown.
But now I must tell you the honest truth:
There is no better snack than plain ole fruit.

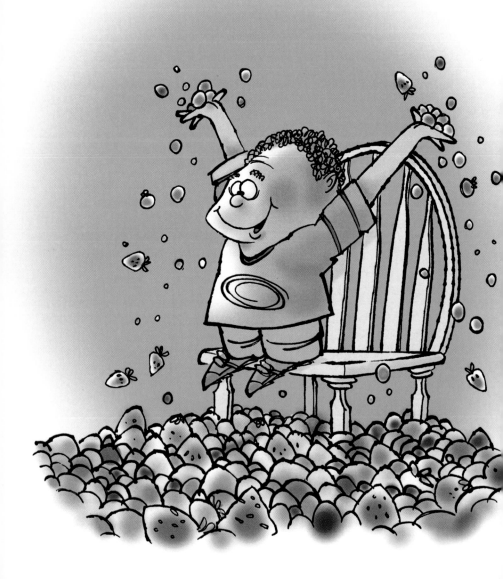

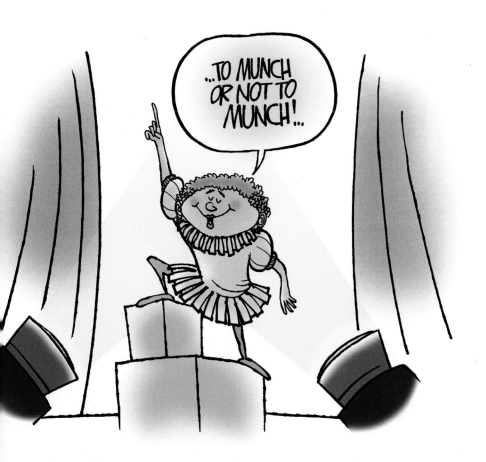

The other day at school, Erica was in a play.
You know how those things are, what they make you say?
Well, it was written by this guy Shakespeare, in olden times,
And she had to talk in strange medieval kinds of rhymes.
It was lunchtime; Erica was hungry and needed to be fed,
When the director pointed to her, this is what she said:

"A Sugar Buster, to be or not to be.
Tis far better to eat right, and I know what is better for me."

Although the play wasn't over, you can guess the rest.
Everyone ran to the cafeteria and chose the food
    that was best.

Jason climbed the stairs to outer space
He sprinted long and won the race
He sailed from here to the seven seas
He swung on the branches of hickory trees.
Today he learned all manner of things in school
     it's plain to see,
But the best time of all was dinner at home with his family.

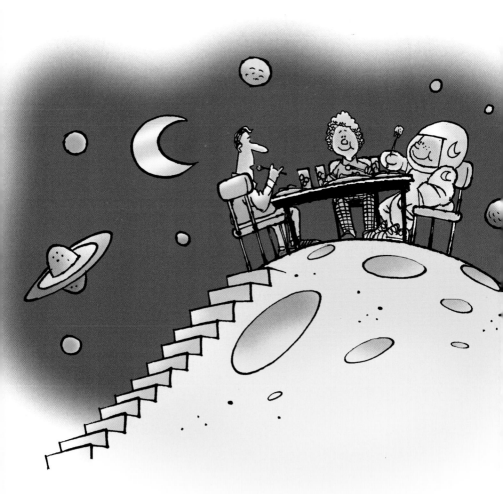

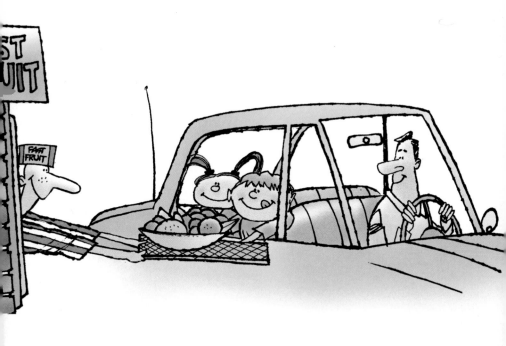

We came in the drive-through round and about,
Came on in this way and drove that way out.
Wanted some fries, burgers, and shakes,
Gave in our order and put on the brakes.
It's quick, oh so quick, but I hope it won't last
'Cause calories, pounds, and indigestion come on so fast.
Wouldn't it, oh wouldn't it be just sooo great
    if they served veggies and fruit,
Then we wouldn't gain so much weight!